Broadening the Circle

Broadening the Circle

The Formative Years and the Future of The Voice Foundation

Martha Howe

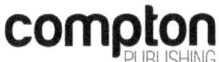

This edition first published 2015 © 2015 by Compton Publishing Ltd.

Registered office: Compton Publishing Ltd, 30 St. Giles', Oxford, OX1 3LE, UK Registered company number: 07831037

Editorial offices: 3 Wrafton Road, Braunton, EX33 2BT, UK
Web: www.comptonpublishing.co.uk

The right of the author to be identified as the author of this work has been asserted in accordance with the UK Copyright, Designs and Patents Act 1988.

All rights reserved. No part of this publication may be reproduced, stored in a retrieval system, or transmitted, in any form or by any means, electronic, mechanical, photocopying, recording or otherwise, except as permitted by the UK Copyright, Designs and Patents Act 1988, without the prior permission of the publisher.

Trademarks: Designations used by companies to distinguish their products are often claimed as trademarks. Any brand names and product names used in this book are trade names, service marks, trademarks or registered trademarks of their respective owners. The publisher is not associated with any product or vendor mentioned in this book.

Disclaimer: This book is designed to provide helpful information on the subject discussed. This book is not meant to be used, nor should it be used, to diagnose or treat any medical condition. For diagnosis or treatment of any medical condition, consult your own physician. The publisher and author are not responsible for any specific medical condition that may require medical supervision and are not liable for any damages or negative consequences to any person reading or following the information in this book. References are provided for informational purposes only and do not constitute endorsement of any product, website, or other source.

Permissions: Where necessary, the publisher and author(s) have made every attempt to contact copyright owners and clear permissions for copyrighted materials. In the event that this has not been possible, the publisher invites the copyright owner to contact them so that the necessary acknowledgments can be made.

PAPERBACK ISBN 978-1-909082-50-2
HARDBACK ISBN 978-1-909082-51-9

A catalogue record for this book is available from the British Library.

Cover design: David Siddall, http://www.davidsiddall.com

Set in 11pt Adobe Caslon Pro/Myriad Pro by Stuart Brown

1   2015

Table of Contents

Raison d'être and Acknowledgments	vii
1 Provenance	1
2 War of the Words	5
3 Early Days	9
Back-Stories: *R.J. Baken, Lucille Rubin, Cynthia Hoffmann, John A. Haskell*	21
4 Master of Mindfulness	25
5 Ripple Effect	31
Back-Stories: *Katherine Ardo, C. Richard Stasney, Gwen Korovin, Ingo Titze, John Rubin*	41
6 Fiberoptics – Getting Behind the Curtain	47
7 The Art of Laryngology ~	53
8 ~ A Surgical Specialty	59
Back-Stories: *Robert T. Sataloff, Linda M. Carroll, William Riley, Mary Hawkshaw*	62
9 Educating Each Other	67
10 Philadelphia	73
11 Balance of Culture and Science	85
Back-Stories: *Johan Sundberg, Raymond H. Colton, Harvey M. Tucker, Ronald C. Scherer*	91
12 Seeing Sound	95
13 Greater Resolution and Precision	101
14 Exploring Beyond Habit	105
Back-Stories: *Bonnie Raphael, Mara Behlau, Harolyn Blackwell, Christine Sapienza*	110
15 Breath – There Be Dragons	115
16 In the Trenches	119
Back-Stories: *Michael Benninger, Jeannette LoVetri, Peak Woo*	126
17 To-Do List	129
18 Outside the Box	135
19 Broadening the Circle	139
Appendices	141
About the Author	147

This book is dedicated to the many people who through the decades have contributed their time, insights, experiences, knowledge, energy, and support to the creation and furtherance of The Voice Foundation.

Raison d'être and Acknowledgments

Late in the 2013 Voice Foundation Symposium, Mary Hawkshaw and Maria Russo were catching their breath in the staff room, and Mary made the observation that only thirty years ago, there were only three doctors' offices in the United States with videostroboscopes. Seeing Maria's and my surprise, she added that the medical textbooks did not yet have chapters on laryngology, and fellowships in laryngology did not yet exist. The first otolaryngology textbook chapter about the care of singers, written by Dr Robert T. Sataloff, was published in 1986. A great deal of ground has been covered since then.

There was a major turning point in voice science, medicine, and pedagogy in the late 1960s when Dr Wilbur James Gould and Dr Hans von Leden decided to gather the best minds in voice science, medicine, speech pathology, and pedagogy together to start Collegium Medicorum Theatri (CoMeT) and The Voice Foundation (TVF). Finding communicative common ground at the early Symposia was an adventure, and involved shouting matches that stopped just short of fisticuffs upon occasion, but there was also tremendous patience and graciousness on all sides. This book is a gathering together of some of those stories.

The perspective is from twenty-four brilliant, generous, leaders in their respective fields, who were attending the Symposia in the formative years, and are a representative mix of speech pathologists, pedagogues, performers, medical doctors, and scientists. It was a privilege and pleasure to speak with them and gather their stories, experiences, and thoughts about Dr Gould, The Voice Foundation, the Symposia, voice science, and what led them to their specialty.

Each interview took five hours or more to transcribe, and when the interview list doubled, TVF Executive Director Maria Russo and the Advisory Board produced six graduate (and beyond) interns and volunteers who transcribed thirteen of the interviews. They saved the day and made the book possible; Carolyn Alexander and Payton Burnette carved out time in their packed semesters for one each, David Young managed two between rotations and applying for a fellowship, and Brock Meadath, Ona Reed, and Nathaniel Sundholm accomplished a remarkable (and deeply appreciated) three each.

After transcribing Mara Behlau's interview, Brock Meadath wrote, "It was extremely enjoyable, she is such a wonderful storyteller! She was actually the primary author on one of my favorite papers in my Voice Disorders: Special Populations course several semesters ago, so it was quite nice to hear more from her." And having transcribed Dr Sataloff's interview, David Young commented: "Such a brilliant and articulate man! I especially liked his thoughts about the future of the field and the sort of paradigm shift that needs to happen. He has such an interesting and fresh perspective. Anytime I listen to him speak or read one of his papers, I come away with a new outlook and new ideas."

Among the many to be thanked, my deepest gratitude goes to the patient and accommodating Noel McPherson of Compton Publishing Ltd, to my insightful soundboards, Tara, Leonore, and Dimaris, for Dimaris' 'perfect grant' question, for Maria Russo's friendship, belief, and multi-level support, Mary Hawkshaw's inspiration, and Dr Sataloff's steady support.

Deepest thanks to the following kind and generous people who took the time from their intense schedules to share their experiences of Dr Gould, The Voice Foundation, the Symposia, and voice science.

Quotes Designation	Full Name
K. Ardo	Katherine Ardo
R. J. Baken, PhD	R. J. Baken, PhD
M. Behlau, PhD	Mara Behlau, PhD, ASHA Fellow
M. Benninger, MD	Michael Benninger, MD, FACS
H. Blackwell	Harolyn Blackwell
L. M. Carroll, CCC-SLP	Linda Carroll, PhD, CCC-SLP, ASHA Fellow
R. H. Colton, PhD	Raymond H. Colton, PhD
J. A. Haskell, CCC-SLP	John A. Haskell, EdD, CCC-SLP
M. Hawkshaw, CORLN	Mary Hawkshaw, BSN, RN, CORLN
C. Hoffmann, PhD	Cynthia Hoffmann, Hon, PhD
G. Korovin, MD	Gwen Korovin, MD
J. LoVetri	Jeannette "Jeanie" LoVetri
B. Raphael, PhD	Bonnie N. Raphael, PhD
W. Riley	William "Bill" Riley
J. Rubin, MD	John Rubin, MD, FACS, FRCS
L. Rubin, PhD	Lucille Rubin, PhD
C. Sapienza, PhD	Christine Sapienza, PhD
R. T. Sataloff, MD, DMA	Robert T. Sataloff, MD, DMA, FACS
R. C. Scherer, PhD	Ronald C. Scherer, PhD, ASHA Fellow
C. R. Stasney, MD	C. Richard Stasney, MD, FACS
J. Sundberg, PhD	Johan Sundberg, PhD
I. Titze, PhD	Ingo Titze, PhD
H. M. Tucker, MD	Harvey M. Tucker, MD, FACS
P. Woo, MD	Peak Woo, MD, FACS

1

Provenance

> Much of what happens in history, I think, is due to the devoted and inspired contribution of single people.
>
> J. Sundberg, PhD

Gathering together voice scientists, laryngologists, voice pedagogues, clinicians, speech-language pathologists, and performers to share their information with each other was a new concept when Dr Wilbur James Gould organized the first 'Care of the Professional Voice' Symposium in 1971. He was determined that the various professions would find a way to communicate with each other, and knew that they would all benefit from the information and insights produced from this exploring of their common ground.

In his Editor's Note to the transcription of the 1978 Symposium, Dr Van L. Lawrence wrote: "The intent of this Symposium is to assist the various disciplines committed to vocal research and voice care, by discussing their shared problems and results, thus helping in the creation of a common language for mutual understanding."

Through interviews with twenty-four of the people who helped form and expand The Voice Foundation Symposia, this book looks at the patience and perseverance of those who were there in the first years, how the cross-hybridization has changed lives and spurred breakthroughs creating a body of literature which in turn promoted further research, and takes a quick look at various research wish-lists along with some of the cutting edge research being done at the time of writing.

Participants return to The Voice Foundation Symposia year after year, from around the world, both because of the warmth and collegiality, and because they are guaranteed to hear the most recent research findings in all the voice professions, along with information on the newest surgical procedures, and lectures by leading voice clinicians demonstrating their most effective methods.

Thirty years ago there were less than a hundred laryngeal stroboscopes in the United States, and it was only twenty years ago that the videostroboscope truly gained in popularity, with the intersection of video and smaller, faster computers. The rapid growth in digital electronics has changed the game for voice science and voice medicine, and the technology continues to advance. Meanwhile, some of the most basic vocal functions remain mysterious, possibly simply waiting for the change in technology that will allow for different, less obtrusive, or more subtle measurements. Several open questions are: Why is there such a disparity between self-perception of tone, vibration, and resonance, and what appears on the scope or is heard by the listener? What physically comprises a good breath or a supported or unsupported tone? Can we find agreement on what particular vocal styles sound like?

These and other yet-unanswered questions were addressed over a century ago by Dr Frank E. Miller, the leading laryngologist in New York City at the time, in his book *The Voice: Its Production, Care and Preservation* in which he addressed the science and the art of singing, and acknowledged the need for a voice-team approach to vocal rehabilitation. (The 1910, sixth edition can be found online through The Project Gutenberg Ebooks.) Dr Miller often references one of the pioneers of laryngology, Sir Morell Mackenzie, through his 1886 book, *The Hygiene of the Vocal Organs: A Practical Handbook for Singers and Speakers* giving a good overview of what was known at the time.

Dr Miller's book demonstrates that over this past century although many questions have been answered, many of the issues, questions, and problems remain. Before launching into a chapter each on the in-breath and the out-breath (still a great unsolved riddle), Dr Miller spends a chapter on "The Choice of a Teacher", writing "All this goes to prove that a method, to be elastic and adaptable, should be based on a knowledge of the physiology of the voice-producing organs . . . ." Excellent advice, and a message that The Voice Foundation is still promoting.

In the 1960s, laryngologists were few and far between in the United States, with many of them having escaped the persecutions of World War II. The primary laryngologists in New York City were Dr Gould, Dr Brodnitz, Dr Grabscheid, and Dr Reckford. These names had legendary status among voice performers, who were often fanatically loyal. There were no fellowships in laryngology, no videostroboscopes, no textbooks, and very little published on professional voice care. The actual structure of the vocal folds was not yet clarified, and instrumentation was basic at best.

The idea for The Voice Foundation originated with Dr W. James Gould, who had a firm belief in cooperation over competition, and that people should communicate with each other. He would regularly get together with the top laryngologists across the United States, among them Dr Hans von Leden, who was born in Poland in 1918. The von Leden family immigrated to the United States in the late 1930s when they saw what was happening politically in Europe. Dr von Leden studied in Chicago, and then focused on otolaryngology and plastic surgery at the Mayo Clinic before becoming a throat specialist in Chicago. An acknowledged expert, sought out by voice professionals, he was a pioneer in the field of microsurgery of the larynx to restore and improve vocal function. His obituary, written by Jürgen Wendler on the CoMeT website, comet-collegium.com, is fascinating reading.

During the 1950s, while tenured at Northwestern University, Dr von Leden created a way to examine patients using a periscope lens and a camera mounted on a helmet that fed to a closed-circuit television.

C. R. Stasney, MD: Hans von Leden had been in Chicago, then he moved to Los Angeles in Beverley Hills, Jim Gould, Friedrich Brodnitz in New York, and Van Lawrence in Houston. They got together to swap stories and compare notes.

The purpose of The Voice Foundation was to add science to what was pretty much an art form. When I first started in voice, there was very little science, and thanks to Titze, Hirano, Gould, and Brodnitz, science was introduced to it, with the caveat from Brodnitz that, "You need to stay holistic, people!"

J. A. Haskell, CCC-SLP: One thing that is interesting in all of this, is not only the change in medicine and exploring the voice, looking at the voice, and listening to the voice, but the difference in practices.

Dr Brodnitz came over from Berlin in 1937, along with other ENTs who were escaping Germany and Austria, and set up a private practice in New York City. In those days, people were mostly solo practitioners. He had an office at Madison and 61st for many years. He may have shared a secretary with other doctors, but they were all separate practices. (I remember watching him type out his own bills.)

I got to know Brodnitz because I heard that he had space in his office when I was looking for an office. I was looking with a colleague, and decided that this was going to be great for us. We took two or three rooms, and there was a large waiting room.

He was a smart, great doctor and a wonderful guy. Video tapes are still available of him demonstrating the chewing method: a method set up by Emil Froeschels, also an immigrant. This is a method for voice therapy that he based on the idea that primitive man could talk and chew at the same time, and if you could do that, like primitive man, your voice would function better. No one really took it seriously other than Froeschels, but the idea was the action of chewing. By working on chewing, and separating it, initially, from content, adding humming, speaking numbers while chewing in an exaggerated way, then calming it down while adding more speech, the voice would improve. It was used for stuttering, all sorts of things, and is still taught in voice disorder classes. I use my own version of it. He was wonderful to listen to, the great old school, as you can imagine, great at presentations, he was so full of life and so full of experience and wisdom.

I didn't work *with* him very much, but we talked about patients and a number of things, and he was a frequent contributor to the Symposia, either demonstrating, or presenting one thing or another. Everybody loved him. He was a very special person.

He worked with a lot of singers, whom I also got to know. Leontyne Price went to see him whenever she had a performance in New York, just to get clearance. He had helped her when she had a vocal breakdown. She was singing *Fanciulla* at the Met and couldn't finish the performance. I think Dorothy Kirsten came in to finish those performances. Brodnitz helped her through this, and helped her figure out that she shouldn't have been singing at that time, because of her menstrual cycle. She had been his patient before, and she loved him. He understood her, worked with her, and talked with her. She trusted him. He really inspired confidence. Very genuine but very strict in his way, with a sense of humor. There were lots of singers and actors who came in; there were pictures of a lot of them on the wall.

That was the time of the solo practitioner, which is rare now. There's more communication, and its different now in the way doctors work together.

R. T. Sataloff, MD, DMA: Von Leden, Brodnitz, and Gould were all involved together in starting The Voice Foundation and were completely supportive of each other's efforts. Gould was involved in CoMeT (Collegium Medicorum Theatri) early on, from the beginning, and von Leden was involved with The Voice Foundation from the beginning.

The organizations just used different approaches, for different purposes. In those days people didn't bother putting that sort of stuff in writing; and they talked to each other (there were no emails).

The Collegium membership has relatively small meetings where we talk with each other. The Voice Foundation Symposia bring in many people from different academic backgrounds and at different levels, so the purposes and the execution are very different but complementary.

J. Rubin, MD: Jim Gould, of course, was a founding member of CoMeT. I believe that it was the fundamental aim of the founders, when they first thought up the idea, to set up an organization that would allow people interested in care of the professional voice from around the world to liaise, meet both professionally and socially, and maintain relationships. I think they were also interested in, if there was, say, an opera singer who was going to be in Vienna, or Leipzig, or San Francisco, or New York, *et cetera*, that if they got into trouble they'd have a cadre of individuals that could help out. I think that was sort of the unwritten idea. It became the Collegium Medicorum Theatri.

Jim, certainly when I knew him, was so enthusiastic about bringing people together, getting people trained, and getting people interested in voice, and he was so excited about multidisciplnary care. To meet him was almost a revelation. So many times I saw a young academic sort of teeter into The Voice Foundation Symposium and he'd meet with Jim and go away all fired up. Jim Gould was an amazing man. He certainly could communicate with people from all walks of life.

Save A Voice Foundation (the name was changed to The Voice Foundation in 1975) and CoMeT were both created in 1969, by laryngologists willing to work together to create a network that would advance vocal science and knowledge. It was known among performers that you could call Dr Gould's office, and his secretary would give you the name of a laryngologist anywhere you might find yourself in the world. This Rolodex helped create CoMeT, which in turn added to the Rolodex of names of those who dealt directly with voice performers and professionals. That famous Rolodex has been replaced by the CoMeT website's membership list. Unfortunately, very few voice professionals know of this website or its list.

Save A Voice Foundation grew out of Dr Gould's vision of interdisciplinary communication, and his desire to do what the title suggests. His charm, ability to communicate easily with everyone, boundless energy, and entrepreneurial outlook coaxed very busy doctors out of their surgeries and private practice offices, voice scientists and their graduate students from their labs, and speech language pathologists, voice pedagogues, and voice performers from their clinics, studios, rehearsals, and classrooms. In 1971, they all started gathering together for Care of the Professional Voice, the first truly interdisciplinary Symposium.

P. Woo, MD: I remember all the big names from that era – those were people who took a lot of effort out of their day and their practice; it was a labor of love. Those people should be given the acknowledgment and the credit for having the vision to come together and push voice science, as well as steer the professional voice forward.

2

War of the Words

I would go to Jim Gould complaining, "This is hopeless. This is just hopeless. We can't even agree on a basic thing. We'll never get anywhere." And Jim would respond, in that calm, quiet, and deliberate way that he had: "We will learn to talk to each other."

R.J. Baken, PhD

P. Woo, MD: At the early Symposia, you had a fairly large number of dramatic personalities. The singers would have their ideas and they would be very vocal in expressing them. There were some singers who felt it was an art form, so why try and understand it? They weren't interested in any kind of science. And there were other singers who felt it should be more scientifically oriented.

I think some of the major physicians of that period of time did steer it towards science; for example Dr Hirano, Dr Sundberg, Dr Brewer, Dr von Leden, Dr Brodnitz, and Dr Moore, were more of the scientific founders of The Voice Foundation. They were the key supporters in those early years in New York.

I remember the brain-storm sessions even after the Symposia with people like Ray Colton, Tom Murray, Paul Moore, we would just sit around and shoot the breeze about things like, we don't really know what causes people to get loud – which part of the vocal folds? It was a good time. We used to sit around and have a beer and talk about all the things we don't know, rather than what we do know.

―――――

B. Raphael, PhD: It seems like some questions never got answered, like at the beginning, we tried, we really did try, to put together a Voice Foundation glossary, with definitions and terms we could agree on. There was a voice teachers' committee, and there was a singing teachers' committee, and there was a doctors' committee, and all these committees with the same list of terms, and we were supposed to come up with our definitions of all these different terms and then come together and agree on them… forget about it, it never happened! We tried for a couple of years and we finally threw up our hands and said, "You know, this is not gonna happen."

―――――

I. Titze, PhD: I first attended a TVF Symposium in 1978. The sessions produced big arguments, ones that took years to settle, especially regarding registers.

We met at Juilliard, mostly discussing registers. There were such emotional outbursts that people got out of their seats and were yelling at each other. I remember Tom Shipp trying to bring the room back to order and saying, "Sit down now! You've spoken enough!" I've since then spent decades trying to figure out what registers are and how to label them. We believe we finally have scientific answers.

J. Sundberg, PhD: People get quite furious about register terminology. It has a very strong emotional loading charge, ah that's funny. As long as you don't know the facts, then you could replace arguments with emotions.

In these next two quotations, Dr Titze and Dr Baken explain beautifully why so much of the early communication was at cross-purposes between the scientists and the clinicians. These elemental differences are still evident and continue to take patience to negotiate, but there is also much more common ground and respect on both sides.

I. Titze, PhD: I enjoyed the interdisciplinary nature of the Symposia, how scientists acted and reacted to clinicians and pedagogues. I recall a participant, Elizabeth Howell, who used to get frustrated and say, "Why don't you scientists ever say what is, or what isn't?! Why do you always qualify everything with 'maybe' and 'probably'?"

Science has to use cautious language. A scientist is taught to give all the conditions and caveats. Science can't prove anything, it can only disprove. We say that we gain confidence as more and more attempts to disprove fail. Teachers and clinicians, however, have to give positive statements or their clients will leave. So they often over-state their point of view. Learning about selling your statements to the other disciplines was a very hard, yet rewarding process. Now, I see more understanding of that process in our Symposia.

R. J. Baken, PhD: I came out of a liberal arts undergraduate program with a degree in romance languages, so I've been on both sides of the arts/humanities vs. the sciences issue. An important difference between C. P. Snow's 'two cultures' [sciences and the humanities] is that the arts continually try to broaden categories. Think of what is meant today by 'symphony' – originally a relatively short musical piece between segments of a larger work. But radically different musical offerings, from Mozart and Haydn, to Stravinsky and Hindemith are all now captured under the 'symphony' heading. A similar tale can be told for the literary class 'novel'. What is a 'novel'? Sterne's *Tristram Shandy* and Robbe-Grillet's *Le voyeur* are both allowed under this rubric. The sciences, on the other hand, constantly try to narrow categories. Scientists expel things from a category to form a new category. One is not allowed to include something under a specific heading unless it meets a strict definition.

Clinicians, performers and teachers are especially prone to using empirical evidence to cement their present knowledge in stone. That's what works, after all, and their clients expect to be given techniques that work. A performer is trained to dive deeply enough into an interpretation that the audience believes it and experiences it as true. However, tomorrow night there may be a different 'truth' to embody. These fundamental differences in viewpoint created a level of distrust, where the scientists felt non-scientists were being erratic, overly emotional and illogical, and the clinicians, performers and teachers felt looked down upon and that their opinions were dismissed and under-valued.

Those who study cultural trends will of course recognize this as one of the pervading cultural conflicts of the twentieth century, especially the second half of it, and it is reassuring that over time in the Symposia a general level of mutual understanding, common purpose, and clear lines of communication have been created and upheld. Dr Gould's vision survived, we did find a way to talk to each other:

R.J. Baken, PhD: My recollection is that we originally drew perhaps a hundred people, if that many. Certainly, in the very first years the Symposium didn't come close to filling even the moderate-sized Paul Hall at The Juilliard School, where we were originally housed.

The first several years of the Symposia were, as I recall, dominated by one question, which provoked often bitter, occasionally ugly, and sometimes recriminative debate. And that was, "What is a register?" There were infinite disagreements and misunderstandings and differences of perspective between what were then two camps, basically the singers and the scientists. For the first four or five years, it seemed to me that every ten minutes a fight over register would break out. I would go to Jim Gould complaining, "This is hopeless. This is just hopeless. We can't even agree on a basic thing. We'll never get anywhere." And Jim would respond, in that calm, quiet, and deliberate way that he had: "We will learn to talk to each other."

While I think the issue of registers has never been resolved, he was quite correct. We *have* learned to talk to each other, and to do so in a reasonable manner with some cognizance on each side of the other side's perspective. I think that today we understand each other's language better, although I don't know that there is necessarily much agreement with some of that language. And I do believe that Jim was correct, we have learned to talk to each other. We have come to understand what the other side means, we have come to understand the opposing perspective. So I think we can have intelligent conversations, if only to disagree, which is something that didn't happen in the old days because we would talk past each other. Now, no matter how wrong-headed I may think others are, I at least understand what they are talking about, and that gives me an opportunity to try to convince them, and them an opportunity to try and convince me.

At the early Symposia there was a clear division into two camps: the singing and the non-singing, the worlds of science and the arts. Each of those has since subdivided, so we now have overlapping groups, different professional constituencies that are easily recognizable. There are, for instance, the surgeons, the physiologists, the engineers, the singers, the non-singing stage performers, the vocal pedagogues, the voice therapists.

In many ways, the professional inclusivity of the Symposia has provided a model for other professional meetings. Most of the work that I do, and the conferences I attend, are outside of the U.S., and I am struck by how many conferences – British Voice Association, Pan-European Voice Conference, Hong Kong Voice Foundation, Collegium Medicorum Theatri – look and feel like the Symposium.

3

Early Days

As long as you don't know the facts, then you could replace arguments with emotions.

J. Sundberg, PhD

R.J. Baken, PhD: There are, to the best of my knowledge, very few records from those first Symposia. (The desire for historical documentation grows only in the light of hindsight.) But there certainly was a lot more informality. I don't recall who made decisions about who was going to present and who wasn't. Somehow, at least from my perspective, it seemed to happen under the radar. I remember chipping in with what needed to be done. What would happen is that Jim Gould would give you a phone call. It was exceedingly hard to say "No" to Jim . . . .

Colleagues would make suggestions for programming along the lines of "So-and-so has been doing some interesting stuff, and we ought to hear about it." I do remember that there would often be themes. The one that sticks most prominently in my mind was a session that was primarily devoted to vibrato, and issues associated with it. (In some sense, this was an extension of the argument about registers.) That sticks in my memory because a lot of very good papers were presented. Some of the research, to the best of my knowledge, never saw the light of day again. There were fewer outlets for publishing in those days.

R.H. Colton, PhD: My major professor at the University of Florida, Harry Hollien, was invited by Jim Gould to come to New York City and talk about the voice for the benefit of the singers in the New York area. Afterwards, he told me it was a very informal setting at Juilliard, with Jim Gould and Harry doing a lot of the talking on that first year of the Symposium. I was invited down to participate in the second year. That was nothing like it is now, let me tell you! Although many of the other new invitees knew their topic, I didn't know what I was going to talk about until we got there that day. I recall talking about the anatomy, physiology, of the strap muscles of the neck. Someone else talked about the internal structure of the larynx, the cartilages, the intrinsic muscles etc. It was all basic information, nothing I had to research, but it was a little frightening to not know what you were going to talk about for twenty minutes or so, until just about an hour before you go on.

There were quite a few people there, most from the New York City area. I remember that there were several physicians there. One was Dr Friedrich Brodnitz, and he was a character. I remember him arguing with various people about various topics on the voice, but he always had excellent comments. There was a lot of give and take during the sessions. People would say something and the topic was opened for discussion for quite a lengthy time.

The audience grew to include singers, speech pathologists, physicians, scientists of all ilks, teachers, and you really were exposed to different points of view, and many times you would argue about things that came down to not understanding what the other person was talking about. Some of the definitions were different. Some of the stuff was, from our point of view unscientific, but not for other people, like singers and voice teachers. It came down to understanding each other's terminology. That took a while.

The results in the long run, maybe five to six years at the most, were that we had a much better understanding of each other, and we could discuss things without arguing about them. It still meant rather lively discussions. I miss those lively discussions now.

From the third year on, things were more planned, with planned presentations by the scientists, or the singers would talk about their areas of interest, so we started to get more and more information. And it still maintained a sense of informality with some good discussions for some years. Of course, you would meet up with people during meals and breaks, and there was a lot of informal discussion, which still exists, over meals and off-campus. It took a while before the researchers, teachers and singers got together and started doing research together. I guess that started happening within about six or seven years after the start of the Symposia.

We were always interested in what makes Pavarotti sound so good. Was it born or made? I began doing some research with Jo Estill, a former singer and singing teacher. She and I did a lot of work together, looking at the different mechanisms of different types of singing. What is characteristic of opera, or lieder, or country-western type singing? We began to research these singing styles from various perspectives. I was interested in voice quality: how do you produce that characteristic sound of classical singing or country western? Why does it sound that way? They are still looking at that. Voice quality has been my main interest.

We did our work with voice modes, which are our designations for major quality areas. We found that the vocal tract itself, the resonator part, plays an important role in determining that quality. I should have found it much earlier, as the vocal tract determines vowels as well as consonants, so why wouldn't it affect this too? We started looking at what the vocal tract was doing, not just what the vocal folds were doing.

It wasn't too soon after we began our research that Johan Sundberg started talking about the singers' formant, which is a unique resonance phenomenon. And so we started to look at that, and looked at what the sound source was producing. What kind of a sound are the vocal folds producing, separate from the resonator? Trying to sort that out.

L. Rubin, PhD: The Voice Foundation was small when it started, so the group felt like an enlarged family. The smaller audience of the initial Symposia was great, and microphones were not always necessary as we were in a small theater within The Juilliard School. Everyone attended all sessions. This was a sympatico group, sharing and learning from each other. Panel discussions followed almost every session and audience participation was frequent. I served on many of those panels and found them highly informative.

What I learned from these beginning Symposia was how to find the ring in my voice, get a clean tone, reach high volume levels safely, identify glottal attacks, keep my voice healthy – and a lot about the anatomy and physiology of the voice. Jim taught me to use the incentive spirometer to help my actors avoid glottal attacks and improve breath management.

Many of my questions were answered through presentations made at the Symposia. It also made me address anatomy and physiology in my teaching and training. Once I saw the videos of the voice in action, the scales dropped from my eyes.

Although the first Symposia were recorded, there was no one to transcribe them. During a panel discussion of Projects for the Future on the final day of the Sixth Symposium in 1977, Dr Van Lawrence commented: "In February when Dr Gould came to Houston for our Voice Conference there, I asked him what had become of the reels, the miles and miles and miles of tape that had been made at all of the Symposia that I had attended here. He said that as of that particular time he had been unsuccessful in getting them together in a cohesive form so that they could be published. And I said, foolishly I think, that I would volunteer to try to undertake it for this particular Symposium." And from his Editor's Notes; "I have attempted to give a tracing of the proceedings rather than a literal transcript of the week." Dr Lawrence kindly continued to oversee the transcription of the Symposia tapes for a decade until the inception of the *Journal of Singing*.

Some of the comments from this 1977 panel discussion on Projects for the Future follow.

John Michel, PhD: I think it should be up to the artist, that we want the artist, the vocal teacher, both in singing and in acting now to show us what they do. [...] What were you wanting to accomplish and why did you have them perform a certain act, as opposed to anything else?

David Brewer, MD: I have a feeling that perhaps some of the speakers and perhaps some of the participants would benefit from ideograms of themselves and also particularly some voice and speech training themselves. [...] there are ways of improving our methods of presentation.

Gordon Schaye, MD: I think we have neglected the problems of the school speech teacher. [...] I think it is really pertinent. Also, the geriatric patient. [...] The problem of reconstruction of the larynx also, the pathologically involved larynx [...] those are some of the areas that I think it would be good to consider.

Harry Hollien, PhD: Each presenter in the scientific portion in the first couple of days will be required not only to do a little more term defining, but also relate his work to something useful. After all, scientists don't always remember that they have an obligation to be useful in this world.

Wilbur James Gould, MD: I think we learned something about putting all the scientists off in a corner and having them speak in pure jargon. I don't think we were communicating as well as we could have [...] I am sure you were not saying that there was no interaction, because there was plenty.

Hans von Leden, MD: I wonder if it isn't possible to require of each speaker to present a short summary of his remarks in easily understandable language? That would mean that the physician tries to speak as a non-medical person, and the scientist tries to speak as a non-scientist. In other words, trying to explain what you are going to say to someone whom you might meet casually, or socially. I think there is still considerable difficulty in this process of communication, and I think much of that lies within the speaker, rather than with the audience.

Dr Gould's driving concept that diversifying the audience would ultimately promote better understanding and greater clarity and precision in the various forms of vocal research has proven true over time. It is also supported in contemporary research on the effects of gender and race diversity in science, as summarized in

Katherine W. Phillips' article 'How Diversity Works', (*Scientific American*, October 2014, p.44): "The fact is that if you want to build teams or organizations capable of innovating, you need diversity. Diversity enhances creativity. It encourages the search for novel information and perspectives."

H.M. Tucker, MD: I started attending with the second or third Symposium, and it was a time when the voice was not very high on anybody's radar. We were mainly interested in detecting and curing people with cancer and doing it in ways that would not leave them with no functioning larynx.

The larynx has three important functions: The first and most important is getting air in and out. The second, which is almost as important, is being able to prevent stuff from getting into your wind pipe that shouldn't be there while you swallow, which you do two thousand times every day, not counting when you eat or drink. Every one of those swallows has the potential to have you aspirate, and if that happens often enough, you die of pulmonary complications. Last but not least is voice. The ability to use the voice to communicate is the most recent, phylogenetically, that is, say, evolutionarily.

For humans of course, it has gained tremendous importance, much more so than in probably any other species. All of us in those days, we were interested in voice, but we were satisfied if we could preserve any kind of voice so that the patient could at least speak. Which is of course very important. That is where I came from.

Then I went to this Symposium for the first time, with other disciplines like Speech-Language Pathology, or Voice Therapy. And not only that, they had voice teachers and they had non-medical people who were interested in voice, and they all came together. This was unique, that they brought all of these disciplines together in one place at one time to talk about voice, and it was there that I first began to get interested in voice coaches and the use of the professional voice. I had published a few papers on vocal fold paralysis which is a killer to somebody who depends on their voice for a living, whether it be as an opera singer, god forbid, or even just a lawyer, or a used car salesman, or a preacher for example . . . all of these people need a functioning voice and the closer you can get it to a normal voice the more valuable it's going to be to them, so I have stayed interested because of that.

M. Behlau, PhD: Of course, in the first years we were fifty, eighty, less than one hundred, just one room, so it was cozy. You were there. The dinner was at Tavern on the Green in Central Park, with Professor Minoru Hirano singing. So we had such a special, special opportunity in those times.

I adored when we had a single room, that we could see it all, not running from Room A to Room B. I like the real multidisciplnary approach and that the Symposium is a week-long Symposium. I love that, because you sit there, you meet friends, and then you exchange. And I liked in the past when we had more case presentations than today. I believe that panel discussions with cases: surgical cases, rehabilitation cases, pedagogic cases were wonderful to really help the newcomers in the field to develop skills.

C. Hoffmann, PhD: It was a 'heady' time, especially for a young voice teacher, having the exposure and interaction with expert participants on various aspects of the voice. I became a demonstrating teacher in the vocal workshops (I remember giving a lesson to Ingo Titze) and a member of a number of discussion panels. I also presented a paper on the strap muscles of the larynx, and one with Dr Thomas Hixon on the breathing techniques of opera singers. Dr Gould mentioned that he knew the coming together of so many different aspects of the voice could be difficult in the beginning as we all spoke 'different languages' regarding our various disciplines. However, he felt that this exchange would enhance communication between the disciplines, as well as aid education and future research – which has come to pass thanks to his vision and leadership.

I was impressed by the generosity of my vocal colleagues and others with their willingness to exchange information. We often discussed various seminars and how they related to our individual fields. It was an open, enthusiastic atmosphere where discussions were informal and in the context of the programs. The 'languages' did become more understandable and integrated as the Symposia continued.

Over the years I took home a wealth of information: voice science, information and discussion on vocal registers, information from the various workshops, the breathing project with Dr Hixon and important information gathered there, Johan Sundberg's vocal research and voice modeling, the presentations on vocal health and vocal disorders, TMJ, use of the speaking voice, and the reinforcement of information given by experts in their fields.

I remember even back then it was hard to keep people in the room for the interdisciplinary talks! I took copious notes on subjects that were unfamiliar – at first trying to absorb and understand, then with greater exposure, being better able to absorb and understand.

R.C. Scherer, PhD: Well, I quickly realized that Jim Gould held this intense desire for the various disciplines related to voice to work together, to share information, to clarify concepts, and to grow or develop further, relative to research and application. And it was a perfect match to my own desires and orientation. So from the get-go it was a perfect match for everything that I held professionally and personally. I was sold right off the bat. I always admired Jim Gould a great deal and tried to learn from him how he dealt with people, accepted them, and included them, which matched my leanings perfectly.

One of my very fond memories of Minoru Hirano at the Symposia is that he would be talking about a project and then he would sit down at the overhead projector with a blank sheet of plastic and colored pens. He would draw the axes, put in the data, and show the relationship of the data from the experiment that he was explaining. That is, he would create the figures using the overhead projector during the talk. It was absolutely wonderful. That's a very fond memory of a superior mind teaching by creating the relationships right there in front of you.

J.A. Haskell, CCC-SLP: Dr Gould liked to get people together and to get communication going among specialists dealing with voice in different ways. The main accomplishment of the early years was getting the different professions to talk to each other. The Symposium established a conference style that has been imitated all over the world . . . in the United States, in Europe, South America, and in Asia.

In the earlier days, there were more demonstrations at the major gatherings. More people brought up singers to demonstrate, or recordings to demonstrate, that type of thing. That doesn't happen as much now.

K. Ardo: In 1979, I was going to be singing in New York and the ear, nose, and throat specialist here in Calgary, Dr William Campbell, said he would like to pay for me to stay an extra week in New York, because he wanted me to attend a conference on the Care of the Professional Voice for him.

When I met Dr Gould, I remembered being treated by him when I was younger, while singing at the University of Toronto. I had been having some difficulties with my voice and nobody could tell us what was going on, neither in Montreal nor in Toronto. It was suggested that I go and see Dr Wilbur James Gould in New York and that he would be the best person to let me know what was going on. And you know, I can't even remember, it might have just been gastric reflux. But at the time, gastric reflux wasn't taken seriously for singers.

So this was a kind of reunion for me to recognize this gentleman after so many years. At the Symposium I was overwhelmed in this room of five hundred participants, most of whom were from everywhere in the world except Canada. There were only three Canadians there. I had worked with some of the best teachers in the world, and after more than ten years singing in West Berlin, I thought I knew everything there was to know about voice until, suddenly, this awakening happened during the Symposium, when I realized I knew nothing about the voice.

And I was thrilled. I was transported, really, into another period of my life. When I got home and told Dr Campbell all about the conference, thanking him extremely for making this revelation possible, I said to him that I thought because of my post-polio difficulties I really wanted to go and study a little bit more.

W. Riley: When The Voice Foundation first began, there were two missions: One was to stimulate and develop new research, and the other to fund new research. It is virtually impossible to get funding for something that is a brand new idea. So one of the missions was to give some seed money for a new idea or a new corporation, or a new perspective. Small grants for researchers were part of our initial work. It had to be novel research – a new idea that would be presented at the Symposia. Much later, because so many foreigners and graduate students were coming, we went through a phase when it became more of a tutorial in voice, speech and research. There are lots of conferences where you can get tutorials about medicine, but this one was really about voice.

R. T. Sataloff, MD, DMA: *When you first started attending the Symposia, what struck you?* The interdisciplinary science and collegiality. The fact that there were not only clinicians, but also researchers with backgrounds in communication disorders, physics, computer science, and other areas that were devoting their professional lives to the human voice, and that they were meeting annually to establish and enhance lines of communication with people in other disciplines like medicine, also interested in voice.

It was a strikingly intellectually energetic gathering of people, and its existence was virtually unknown in academic otolaryngology.

In fact, I had planned to create such an organization, and I was just delighted to find out that I didn't have to because there was one in existence in which my input was welcomed to help enhance and expand it.

Probably the greatest initial opportunities were the interactions with world-class scientists, so that clinical questions could be posed, and researchers would dedicate their time to addressing problems of importance to patients. Within a year or two, answers would be presented at the Symposia, and the next week they would be in offices across the world, making people better before the new information was even published.

There were, of course, clinical advances that were presented that ranged from things that I presented, like micro flap and mini micro flap surgery, and surgical instrumentation, as well as instrumentation and techniques that were presented and developed by Dr Marc Bouchayer in France, early use of video in voice diagnosis and other innovations. All these gave attendees not only things like new instruments, but also new ideas, approaches, and challenges to develop diagnostic refinements.

I. Titze, PhD: The interdisciplinary aspect of the Symposia affected my work enormously. Floods of new thoughts raced through my mind, flying back from the Symposia to Iowa or Denver. Unfortunately, when I got back to my desk and everything was stacked up after a week away, only one or two new thoughts turned into action.

It was funny being in the Mayflower Hotel in New York. I recall many discussions that continued from Lincoln Center into the hallways of the Mayflower Hotel. Often we were engaged with each other all day long. I haven't been in the Mayflower since, but that was the gathering place for many years.

I was one of the Central Park joggers – that was a highlight – luckily we were never bothered by anybody. There were major discussions that took place during those runs.

M. Benninger, MD: When I first went it was a little intimidating. It was at the Juilliard, and I was giving a presentation with dual slide projectors, because that's what we typically did back in those days, and they didn't have the set-up for dual slide projectors so they had me project onto the back wall of the stage. It was towards the end of the program so there weren't a whole lot of people in the audience by that time, although I got to interact a lot with those people beforehand.

I can remember Ron Scherer just asking me these remarkable, specific, questions that I had no idea how to answer. Here I was a third year resident, this is my first major presentation at a meeting and the people that are querying me ask me questions about things that I didn't know as a physician. Although it was embarrassing at the time, it actually stimulated me to try and find the answers. It stimulated me to try to figure out what I do from the perspective of a voice scientist, like Ron. So it actually helped my career rather than hurt it. Then I started going every year.

J. LoVetri: It took me quite a while before I understood enough from the Symposia to have it make a direct impact in what I was doing teaching singing. I would say, what had the most impact were the workshops because there I got to see people work. After watching Lucille Rubin, I had a few sessions with her in New York to understand better what she was doing with speech. That was very useful.

I would go to the workshops and see how different senior teachers were working with students. At that time it was only classical teachers, except for a man named Joe Scott, who had a lot of Broadway students (I think his most famous student was Lainie Kazan). Joe was a good friend of Dr Gould and presented Broadway workshops while we met at Juilliard, but the rest of the faculty was classical.

By 1987, I realized that the world of commercial music, which at that time we called pop music or popular music, was being neglected at the Symposia. I started asking researchers early on, "Do you ever study other styles besides classical?" and was told "No" more times than I care to remember. At that point, the only person who ever presented any information on music that wasn't classical was Jo Estill, who was doing her work on belting. I remember even at the very beginning that I was delighted that somebody was presenting anything that wasn't classical!

I had been teaching Broadway belters since 1980, and really wanted Ms Estill's work to be up there because she was doing something that represented what I did. Unfortunately, when I heard her examples I didn't like the sound she called belting. I didn't recognize it.

My role models were Angela Lansbury and Ethel Merman in her young days, or anybody else who had been on Broadway who produced a traditional belting sound prior to rock and roll. Those women sounded like they were singing and not shrieking. The research presented at that time, on belting, did not seem to me to match the sounds made by these great singers and I was disappointed that the examples presented were not more in keeping with Broadway's expectations and criteria.

At about that same time, I was able to approach Dr Sataloff, who seemed a little less intimidating to me than Dr Gould, since we were the same age, and stated, "If there is any room, I really would love at some time to do a workshop on Broadway singing."

I was invited by Dr Sataloff to teach a workshop on music theater singing training in 1988. After that workshop, Johan Sundberg commented, "I've never seen anybody go from belting to classical sounds to 'mixing.' I think this is fascinating. If you ever are in Sweden, I would love for you to come to the lab and let me see what it is you're doing."

That Fall, in Sweden, Dr Patricia Gramming and Dr Sundberg did research on my vocal production. They spent all day, every day for five days, looking into my throat and having me sing. Then they analyzed what they observed. Once I actually saw what was going on in my throat I was able to make the connections, and I was no longer guessing what was happening. I knew what was happening because I saw it. I saw it. I had the data to prove that I was doing what I said I was doing! And that was very, very, valuable to me because the subjective experience became a re-enforcement of the objective knowledge I had gotten by watching what was going on in my own throat.

It also clarified for me the enormous amount of confusion that people have when they haven't had that experience, which, back then, was still a rare thing.

All of the lectures and presentations of the continually expanding Symposia were fully recorded on reel-to-reel by Anthony Lambiase. These tapes were sent to Houston, where Dr Lawrence's staff would try and make sense of the conversations and debates. The single Transcript was quickly divided into two or three parts, depending on the presentations, and with the growth of the Symposia the Transcripts more than tripled in size through the decade. The information being presented at the Symposia deserved being published, and at that time there were limited opportunities.

L. Carroll, CCC-SLP: The *Journal of Voice* came out of the transcripts from The Voice Foundation Symposia, when Dr Van Lawrence said that he thought he would not have the time or the support staff to continue to transcribe the volumes and volumes of tapes. Suffice it to say, sometimes the credit would be mis-assigned because of some of the participants not being able to be properly identified.

Bob Sataloff was already heavily involved with ENT journals. They decided to turn it into a journal that people could subscribe to, with the income going toward The Voice Foundation, and it would be a scholarly publication where people could get credit for the papers presented. Then they could publish in a peer review journal, with peer reviewers who were highly skilled and really dug into the literature in a time of no internet.

Jim Gould thought that since Bob Sataloff had a bigger staff in Philadelphia and was younger, that it made sense to go ahead with the move to creating the *Journal of Voice*. There was not even a year's gap – the last Symposium Transcript was in 1985, and the 1986 Symposium was the source of the first *Journal of Voice* in 1987, published with Raven Press. Vol. 1 #1. We had decided it would be an incredible issue, setting the standard for what was really important in this field.

W. Riley: Dr Gould and Dr Sataloff had a dedicated, private line. Gould's office had two dedicated lines that no one in the laryngology office was allowed to use. One was a line to the Recording and Research Center of the Denver Center for the Performing Arts (later the National Center for Voice and Speech), and the other one was to The Voice Foundation in Philadelphia. He made a daily call to Denver talking to Dr Ingo Titze about research and how the Recording and Research Center was communicating with NIH, and he'd also make a daily call to Dr Sataloff where they would talk about The Voice Foundation and other things in their lives.

L. Carroll, CCC-SLP and **W. Riley**: John Michel and Bob Coleman used to do 'the dog and pony show', the night before the Symposium fully started – an overview of the physiology of voice and the anatomy. It was always a lot of fun.

What made the Symposia so amazing, especially in New York, was that everything was emerging. It was a completely open forum where you could stand up and either command or take the floor, whether you were a researcher, a physician, a voice teacher, an actor, a singer, a speech pathologist, anything. We'd now gotten to the point where we all knew much more about the physiology of elite voice function and voice teachers were no longer uninformed, so they felt like they were really a part of this collective medical circle. And they were. So The Voice Foundation was unique in that it started with physicians and researchers trying to embrace speech pathologists and the singing community. Then it evolved into a dominance of the speech pathology community, and now it is coming around to where there are more physicians coming back to TVF. It's been an interesting ride. Today when I come to the Symposia, I still remember the old days.

There were six to eight hundred at those Symposia. In New York, it was easier for people to just drop by. We would have our banquet in the lobby area outside Paul Hall, with a small concert for the Faculty people.

New York Galas

L. Carroll, CCC-SLP: Voices of Spring was an annual fundraiser at the beginning of spring, around March 1st, and Gould would bring in a quarter to a half-million dollars. He was very skilled at getting people to write a check. He'd call IBM or Amerati and Hess and ask, "Will you be buying two or three tables?" Each table was ten dinners!

_____

W. Riley: Gould was friends with Anna Moffo who had recorded this fabulous operetta concert piece by Johann Strauss, Voices of Spring, and Gould thought this was the perfect song to characterize the Gala, and in one of the earlier fundraisers he had Anna Moffo sing it. She sang for a lot of the fundraisers. Dr Gould would open up his Rolodex, and he was very good at fund raising. Every year he would do this springtime fundraiser, either at the Waldorf Astoria or the Pierre, and you would be sitting next to celebrities and political personalities. Gould was JFK's college roommate. That's why he was on the campaign trail with JFK, and White House doctor for JFK and LBJ, almost weekly.

Voices of Spring was a big New York society fundraising event, with hundreds of people dressing up to the hilt. They would hear a concert or a masterclass, so they could hear the art that they were supporting, and then hear a short overview lecture of the new medical information from the year so they could hear what their support had helped fund. I remember one presentation on being able to see the vocal folds. The people who would come there were from all walks of life. You'd see the high-powered Wall Street people, and you'd see a 'who's who' from the networks, Broadway stars, and several Metropolitan Opera stars.

_____

H. Blackwell: I performed at only one Gala, which was at the Waldorf Astoria. I had a fantastic time. It was a brilliant evening honoring Anna Moffo, Dan Rather, and Anthony Quinn. There was a tribute to Dr Gould and to each of the awardees. It was very warm and generous, showy and brilliant, all at the same time – everyone was having a wonderful time. It was Mr. Leon Fassler, who I believe was president of the Board at that particular time, who asked me to sing. I knew him from the Opera Orchestra of New York. There was dinner, I entertained and afterwards, we danced the night away. It was a magical night for me.

_____

L. Rubin, PhD: The galas were such fun! Jim made it a point to go around to each table and ask if we were having a good time. He had a wide smile and a word of praise for each of us and he enjoyed taking photos of everyone. I especially enjoyed Dr Hirano (senior) and Joe Estill singing an operatic duet – they brought the house down! As the Gala grew in size we moved into the St. Regis Ballroom. The size of Jim Gould's fan club had grown tremendously!

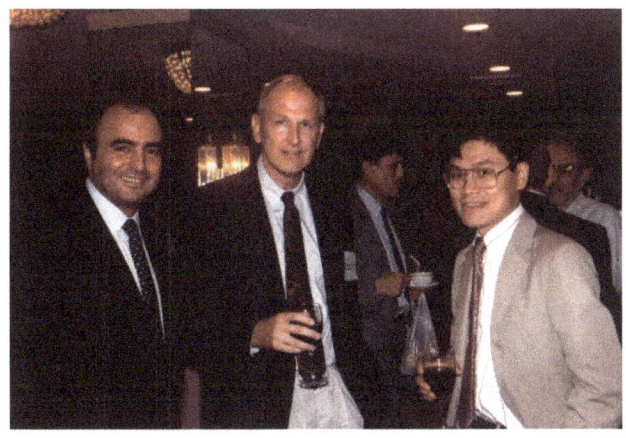

Jean Abitbol, Peter Alberti, Peak Woo

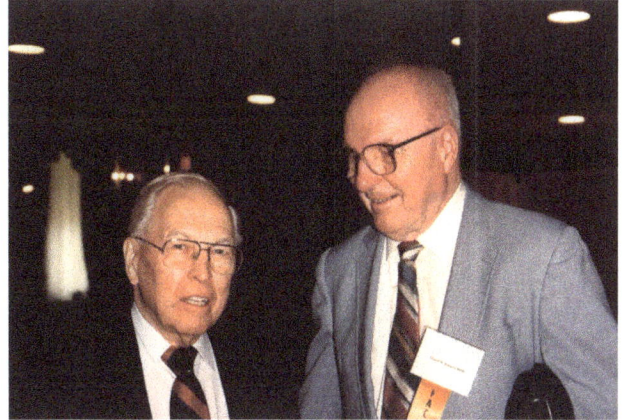

G. Paul Moore, David Brewer

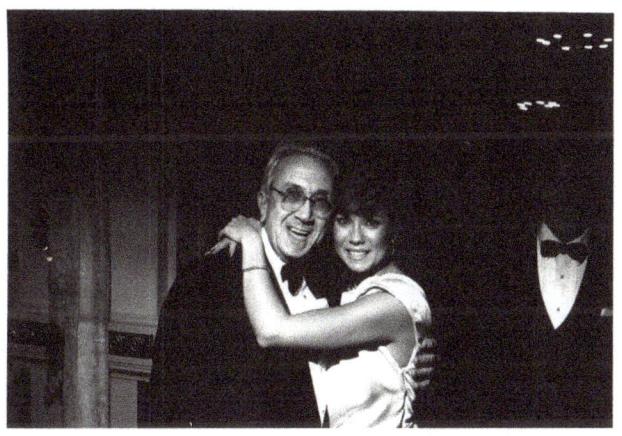

Wilbur James Gould, Kathy Lee Gifford (with Frank Gifford in background)

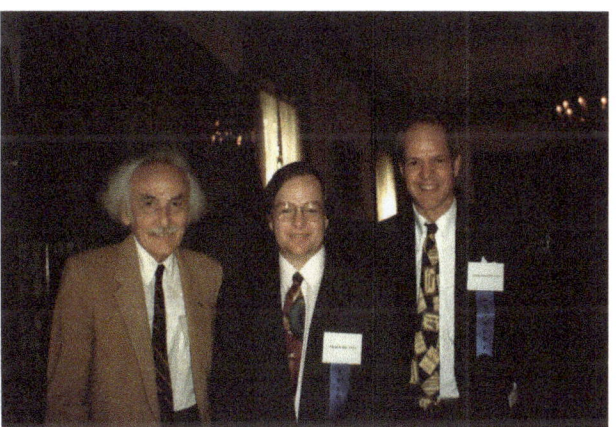

Hans von Leden, William Riley, Richard Stasney

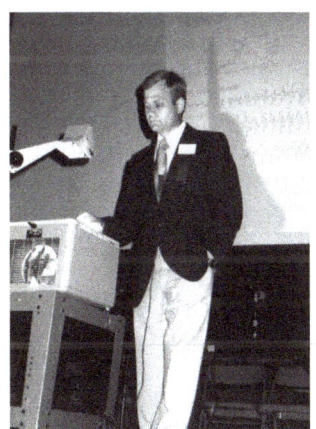

Ingo Titze

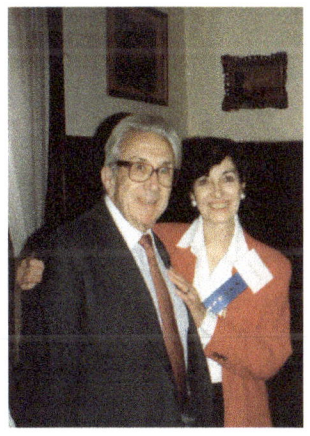

Wilbur James Gould, Lucille Rubin

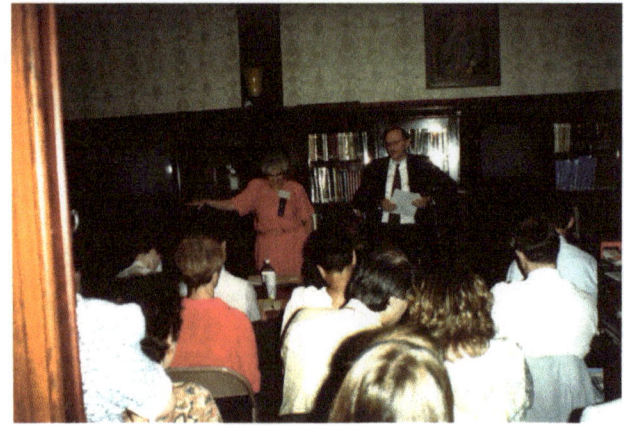
Janina Casper, Ray Colton

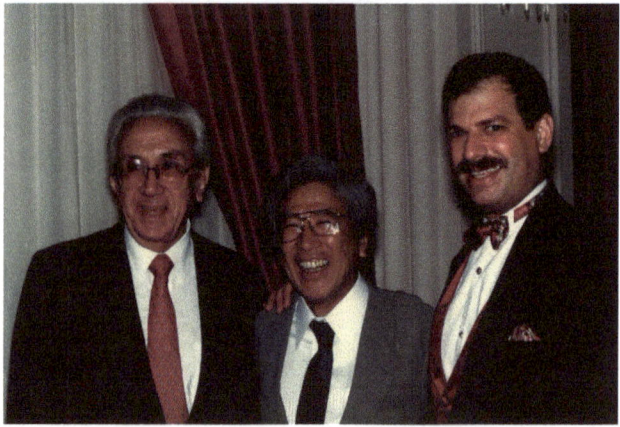
Wilbur James Gould, Shigeru Hirano, Robert T. Sataloff

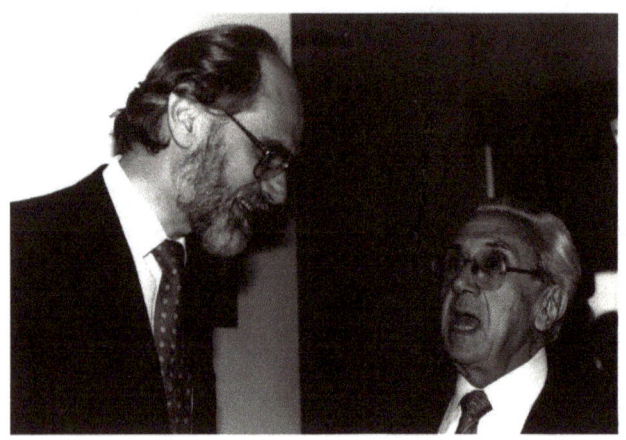
Johan Sundberg, Wilbur James Gould

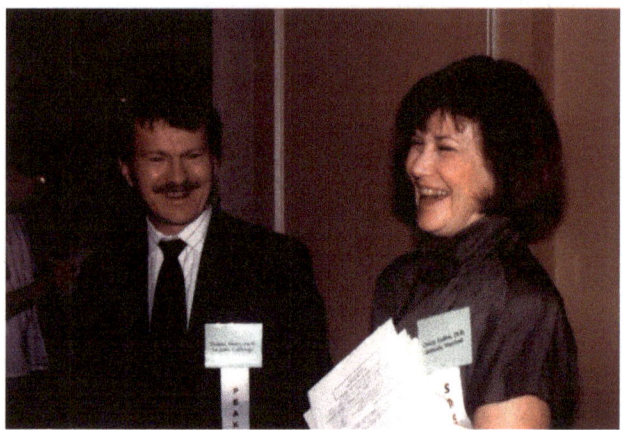
Thomas Murry, Christy Ludlow

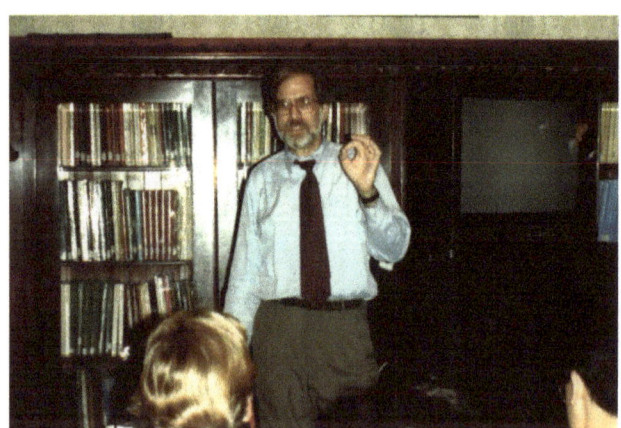
John Haskell

Back-Stories: *R. J. Baken, Lucille Rubin, Cynthia Hoffmann, John A. Haskell*

R. J. Baken, PhD

Director of Laryngology Research, and Co-Chair, Institutional Review Board:
New York Eye and Ear Infirmary of Mount Sinai
Adjunct Professor of Otolaryngology: New York Medical College
Senior Lecturer: New York Medical College, School of Public Health
Professor Emeritus of Speech Science: Columbia University

For my undergrad at Columbia I did a degree in romance languages with a special focus on Middle French. It was an unusual choice; even some of my professors thought I was a little crazy. (Or a lot crazy.) But Columbia College believed that the undergraduate mission is education, as opposed to vocational training, and so they essentially forbade you to study anything that was too useful, but rather encouraged you to pursue your intellectual interests without regard for what that might mean vocationally. So I was a pre-med student, specializing in romance languages, especially medieval. Although I was pre-med I had decided very early on that medicine was not going to be for me, for a lot of reasons.

At one point, I took a course in English phonetics and the instructor intrigued me with a number of questions about general issues of speech production. Given my prior inclination for the medically related sciences, I got deeper and deeper, through a process of slow drift, into larynx and voice production as a chief interest. After my A.B. I went off to do a Masters in speech pathology, and when I finished that I lucked out: Columbia was forming a new department of speech pathology. I studied speech science in that new department and at Columbia's medical school and, while a doctoral student, taught undergraduate phonetics courses. About the time I was finishing my doctorate the speech path department decided they wanted a professor of speech science, and since I was already working on campus, I suppose they just found it convenient to hire me. That was in 1968, and I stayed in the professor biz at Columbia until 1996, when I left to join the 'real world' as the physiologist in the Department of Otolaryngology at the New York Eye and Ear Infirmary. I finally retired in 2003.

Lucille S. Rubin, PhD

CEO: Professionally Speaking New York
Faculty: Circle in the Square Theatre School
Co-Founder: Voice And Speech Trainers Association (VASTA)

I caught the theater bug early – in grade school. I recited poetry in a contest and won, sang in an operetta, and wrote short plays so I could act in them. In High School I was cast in lead roles, and then in college I majored in acting and oral interpretation and also earned a teaching certificate. After graduation, I taught drama and public speaking to high school students. Next was an MA at Northwestern University in both speech and drama, where I met and married my professor who whisked me off to Stanford University where he was finishing his PhD and I took advantage of their theater classes.

The big move was to New York which proved to be a mind-blowing introduction to Broadway shows. I immediately got a job at a modeling school where I taught voice, speech and self-presentation, and also did some fashion runway modeling in large NYC hotels. This was a learning experience but it was time, after raising two children, to get serious about getting a PhD at NYU in theatre acting. Midway, a surprise surgery for a parotid tumor changed my career plans from acting to voice training. This was a eureka moment for me. As the surgery healed, I completed my dissertation entitled 'Voices of the Past: David Garrick, John Philip Kemble and Edmund Kean.'

I settled into the theater department at SUNY Purchase, teaching voice to actors, and on my sabbatical wrote a study on British voice training schools. I also studied, taught and presented in Prague, Moscow, Tokyo, London, Berlin and other cities in the US and abroad. Meanwhile, I was getting requests to coach business professionals, public speakers and working actors so I set up an office in NYC for weekend clients. Soon after, I was approached to teach at Circle in the Square Theatre School, took the job and opened my private practice, Professionally Speaking, in NYC.

While president of University and College Theatre Association (UCTA), I was one of the five founding members of the Voice And Speech Trainers Association (VASTA). I had been actively seeking diverse voice training methodologies that I thought would help VASTA extend its work in the US and abroad. After all this study, training, traveling and degrees, I still had questions that were never answered. So I sought out medical schools that would allow me to sit in on sessions dealing with the voice. Teaching through imagery and sense memory was helpful, but I needed information on the anatomy and physiology of the voice. Scoping at this time was not a reality! I had questions that needed answers. So, I sought out a voice doctor, the world famous ENT, Dr James Gould.

I met with him in his office and asked if I could audit his medical voice lectures at Lenox Hill Hospital. He encouraged me to wait as he was putting together an organization, The Voice Foundation, that would address diverse vocal disciplines: vocal science, medicine & surgery, speech therapy, speaking voice trainers and singing voice teachers.

I could not have designed a better mentor than Jim. He was generous with his time. I gave him a copy of my The Voice Handbook, used by my students and clients, and asked for his feedback. He must have read every word as his feedback was enormously helpful, with specific comments.

Cynthia Hoffmann, PhD

Voice Faculty: The Juilliard School (Chair, Voice Department 1995–2006)
Voice Faculty: Manhattan School of Music

I became interested in vocal pedagogy as an undergraduate voice major, and was encouraged to write an honors project dealing with this subject (which included reference materials such as The Voice of the Mind, by E. Herbert Caesari and Singing, the Mechanism and the Technique, by William Vennard). After graduation, I traveled to New York City to study with my college teacher, Larra Browning, who had also moved to New York and was teaching at the Manhattan School of Music. She had to leave in mid-Spring because of family illness, and asked that I be permitted to teach her pre-college students until her return. Daniel Ferro, Voice Chair, was my supervisor and supported my being able to continue teaching students in the Preparatory Division of MSM when she did not return. This is how I began my teaching career.

When The Voice Foundation Symposia were getting started, Dr Gould was my ENT and mentioned to Oren Brown that he felt it was important to interest young voice teachers and singers in this program because they would bring new ideas and questions into the discussions. He wanted young teachers involved in this interdisciplinary mix as the Symposia moved into the future. Dr Gould was the consummate professional; thorough, informative and personal. His contributions to the voice through his work with The Voice Foundation and Symposia cannot be overstated.

John A. Haskell, CCC-SLP, EdD

Board Recognized Specialist in Fluency Disorders
Co-founder, Co-director: New York City Voice Study Group

Musical comedy was what I wanted as a kid, and I grew up with the great musicals as they were appearing on the scene. It was a pretty exciting period, if you think about it – a great period. So that's what I wanted. In college, I was a theatre and music major and, for a number of years afterwards, I tried to get into the theatre business as a song writer. It's one thing to write musical comedies when you are in college, it's another thing to write them when you are not in college. I'm a pianist, so I coached singers and played auditions. I liked the process of working with singers, so when my father suggested I consider the field of speech pathology I took a couple of courses and decided to continue. I eventually got my Masters and doctoral degrees, and focused on voice as an area of specialization ... one of two areas I specialize in, voice and stuttering.

I had been practicing in NYC since the early 1980s, and don't remember how Dr Gould heard about me. I'm not sure that I had met him before I got the call to visit him in his office. He wanted speech pathologists to whom he could refer patients and, at that time, there were very few people in the city who specialized in voice. We had a very good relationship. I would go see him periodically, say every six months, and we would have a review of patients, go through the files, and I would keep him up to date on everybody.

I continue to play the piano and play chamber music now, playing regularly with a violinist, which is very rewarding. From time to time we play with a cellist, or whoever we can get to play with us. We get together for two hours every Sunday. Right now we're doing Brahms sonatas. We've done a bunch of Beethoven sonatas and Mozart.

4

Master of Mindfulness

Jim Gould was a person who could make himself small in front of large personalities. He got a lot of people to listen to him, and he listened very well himself.

I. Titze, PhD

He was almost a chameleon. He was able to deal with all these different performers on different levels.

G. Korovin, MD

M. Behlau, PhD: Professor Gould was adorable: he was a gentleman, he was so serene, so easy going, particularly with foreigners, and particularly with the newcomers. He had the unique ability of making us feel at home, of softening the heavy stuff. For example, when he was dealing with a patient, if it was a singer with vocal fold nodules, he was not saying that those were nodules, but that this is a kind of adaptation due to the overload you do in your profession, 'simply singing nodes.' He was so careful with words. He had the unique talent of not harming the other's ears, he was careful. He was not . . . because Americans are very assertive to Latin ears. Sometimes we say, "Wow, that was too strong. That was too abrasive. That was too focused, too right to the point." And Professor Gould, he had this unique way of softening the language so you could hear anything from him because he was always going to say it in a very nice manner and you were going to understand.

C. R. Stasney, MD: What an extraordinary man. And he had a nurse who was the go-to person for the entire world. If you were in Addis Ababa or Cairo and needed a laryngologist, everyone called her for a name. She was the encyclopedia for laryngologists in the world.

Jim Gould told me that he had taken care of at least twenty-five sopranos at the Metropolitan opera who had 'singers' calluses.' He would never scare them with the term 'nodules'.

G. Korovin, MD: Dr Gould cultivated the whole voice/laryngology thing. His mother was a physician, an internist/gynecologist, his sister was a physician, an allergist, and her husband was a pediatrician. I think in the very early days, Gould and his sister practiced together a little bit. They took care of a lot of celebrities, so they always came across as coming from a well-connected background, and having a sister and brother-in-law in the medical field who were referring patients to him helped.

He also did some of his early work at Juilliard, working with some of the voice teachers there. In those days Dr Gould, Dr Brodnitz, Dr Grabscheid, and Dr Reckford were the four go-to laryngologists. The other three were old-world German and Austrian.

I swear I remember him telling me he was roommates in college with JFK, and he helped Gould. When JFK was having some voice issues related to his Addison's, he came to Dr Gould and Gould got him through the debates, so his name was out there as being hooked up with JFK.

J. Rubin, MD: He was always early. No matter how early you got to one of his power breakfasts at the Carlyle, he would be sitting at the table. He was a very magnetic individual.

'Mindfulness' implies the ability to be present in the moment, actively observing your thoughts and feelings and what is going on around you without value judgments. It requires setting your ego and sense of self-importance aside, allowing you to react directly, appropriately and cleanly to what is in front of you. This is the quality that kept arising in everyone's recollections about Dr Gould. Forty patients every day, each one feeling completely heard, and he is still the first one at his power breakfasts at 6am or his Thursday teas at 4pm. Anyone who has attempted to practice mindfulness knows how difficult it is, and anyone who has been around a truly mindful person knows what a force of nature they are.

Dr Wilbur James Gould graduated from Harvard in 1941, and New York University Medical School three years later, then he served as a Captain in the United States Army Medical Corps. He was on the faculties of New York University, Columbia University and New York Medical College, and an adviser to the National Institutes of Health, eventually getting them to take voice seriously as a separate category.

In the excellent obituary for Dr Gould, written by Dr R.T. Sataloff in 1994, he notes: "First and foremost, he was a devoted clinician. He was always available to his patients for medical care or wise support, and he routinely made house calls and backstage visits not only for his famous patients, but graciously for anyone. Jim remained as devoted to the most unknown students as he did to his most famous patients, who included such dignitaries as Dwight D. Eisenhower, John F. Kennedy (with whom he traveled), Lyndon Baines Johnson (on whom he operated), President Bill Clinton, Frank Sinatra, Luciano Pavarotti, Mick Jagger, Elizabeth Taylor, Linda Rondstadt, Robert Kennedy, Laurence Rockefeller, Dan Rather, Angela Lansbury, and many others who have come forward to express sorrow at this passing. Nothing was ever more important to him than the health and happiness of his patients."

What was it like sharing office space with Dr Gould?

G. Korovin, MD: He was very welcoming, he would bring me in if there was an interesting patient that he thought I should meet, or be involved with their care, even if I was in another room with my own patients, so I could meet them. So he was very enthusiastic about having me there.

The stroboscope was fascinating to me. I would come in, and he was a master of inserting the flexible stroboscope and doing it. There were people who would say that they'd been at so-and-so's office, who couldn't get a good picture, and they'd say,

"Oh you're never going to be able to stick that thing down my throat! I can't do it, I can't do it." Some people, I'd say, "Try it" and for some reason I learned some of the skills, and I can't even tell you just what, but I picked up something from watching him.

W. Riley: The other thing Gould liked was that I was a calming influence on the patients. If he had someone who was a nervous performer, he said, "I want you to put your hands on them, put your hands on their head and hold them steady." Jim Gould was a psychological genius, and patients loved him.

He was unique because his patients were quite varied and, because they were in New York City, they were quite stressed. Jim had this ability to make his patients feel that they were the center of his life. One of the strategies that he would use, was that before he would walk into an exam room, he would take three slow breaths to clear his mind and focus. The patients would, in effect, feel complete confidence. He was never rushed. He had the ability to convince the patient that he spent a lot of time with them, even though it was often only two or three minutes. They were really getting quality time – his undivided attention.

My office in his suite had the separate door for VIPs. The suite was at 47 E. 77th at the corner of Madison, and when you came up to the second floor you could go straight ahead to the door with the plaque, or you could turn right down the corridor to the second door, which was my office (which also housed the TVF files). So when I heard someone knock, I knew it would be someone like Frank Sinatra or Katherine Hepburn – someone who was a VIP. This is not uncommon in laryngology offices. Many of them have a separate entrance that avoids the front office and reception area. Otherwise you have to close several hours early to clear the clients.

L. Carroll, CCC-SLP: I would be outside the room waiting for Bill [Riley] to be through (in the early 1990s), and Jim would sneak into the back corridor and put his ear to the door. He said "I'm listening." I said, "To what?" He replied, "Magic." Then he smiled and walked away.

J. Rubin, MD: Jim was a sculptor. He used to take sculpting classes somewhere on Third Avenue in the low 80s, and one day at the end of clinic he took me along. The people there were very interested in having another surgeon come, and they got me involved. Sculpting and painting have become a very important part of my own life and that's from having been encouraged by Jim to pick up a chisel.

He was working on a lion when I went sculpting with him. I don't think he had finished it by the time he, sadly, passed away. He was working with alabaster and didn't like to use electric tools – he was using a hammer and chisel. Sort of the Michelangelo approach. It was a pretty big piece. I'd say that the lion was, say maybe 24 inches in length, maybe had a 14 inch base, and probably about 16 inches high. It was quite a nice piece he was working on. It might have even been slightly bigger that that . . . it was quite a heavy piece, being alabaster.

In the 1994 obituary, Dr Sataloff noted that Dr Gould was, "... a renowned collector of memorabilia of Admiral Lord Nelson. His collection of Nelson contains a particularly important collection of love letters written by Lord Nelson to Lady Hamilton. Jim also amassed one of the world's great collections of scrimshaw, much of which now resides in the Smithsonian Museum. In addition to his love of scrimshaw, Jim had a passion for the sea in general, and he spent many happy hours with [his wife] Maureen and friends sailing the east coast in his boat Tawney. [...] An outstanding photographer, Jim's extraordinary photograph of John Fitzgerald Kennedy remains among the finest in existence."

B. Raphael, PhD: He was always incredibly busy, he was always multitasking and he was absolutely charming. I already loved him from The Voice Foundation Symposia that I attended, I think I started attending in 1978 but I attended a bunch of the Symposiums before I got this call, "Do you want to work at the Denver Center?" So I already knew him and admired him greatly. He had a great joy; you know, he was a man who was doing what he was put on Earth to do. His license plate said 'voice'.

You would see these wonderful people presenting at the Symposium and Jim Gould would be in the aisle of the theater at Juilliard with his little camera, snapping their picture. Because he was as much in awe of them as I was, he had a huge love for what he was doing and for the field.

M. Hawkshaw, CORLN: I remember an Academy meeting in New Orleans when Bob, Dr Gould and I were having lunch. Bob was giving a lecture on the final day, and Dr Gould asked, "What's Mary going to do?" Bob replied, "Well, she'll just wait 'till I'm done." Dr Gould said, "No, no, no, no, no. I rented a limousine for her, and I hired a driver and he's going to take her on a tour of New Orleans and show her everything." And that's just the kind of man he was, very thoughtful and generous to all. He was just, just amazing.

H. Blackwell: It was around 1985, through Margaret Hoswell, my voice teacher at the time in NYC, who recommended I have a consultation with Dr Gould. He was very lovely, encouraging and supportive. Being a young singer, I needed positive feedback and reassurance concerning my vocal health. He was careful about giving you the information that you needed, and making sure that you were doing things correctly such as saying: maybe steroids are not the best thing for you, but rather vocal rest would be better.

I felt at ease with him because of his supportive personality. He was good at knowing how to treat singers, help calm our fears, and to give us the knowledge we needed in order to comprehend what was happening to our voices at that particular moment.

It was Dr Gould who was monitoring a friend for reflux, when no one had heard about reflux. He went to Dr Gould. Dr Gould sent him to Dr Sataloff, and they found a problem with his sphincter muscle. Eventually, he had to have an operation. It was the first time I had ever heard about reflux and the problems singers have with reflux.

L. Rubin, PhD: He was taking care of the kings and queens, presidents, stage actors, movie stars, opera singers, musical theatre personalities, high priority business executives – and Madame Chiang Kai-Shek [wife of the then President of the Republic of China]! At times, the street on which Jim had his office was closed when high profile clients were in town.

Jim's knowledge of the singing voice was spectacular. He knew the names of the operas, attended opera, and also was familiar with the scores. An opera singer came into his office and after being examined asked if she could sing the next night at the Met. "What are you singing?" he asked. She answered, and he said: "No, let someone cover for you. If you were singing (and he named another opera), I'd have no reservations."

A well known singing teacher came in complaining that he had had a cold that left him with a deep low pitch that he couldn't get out of. Jim looked into his ears and as he slowly removed some wax, the patient's voice ascended into his natural pitch level! "My voice is back. It's a miracle." Yes, Jim was a kind of a miracle man. He was also very good with patients who would present with a lot of neck and or throat tension. As they would complain Jim would say: "Yeah? Tell me a little more about it" as his hands started a smooth, soft massage to the patient's neck and the tension melted away.

I remember the first day I became his patient for a nasal scoping. I sat in the chair while he diverted my attention elsewhere, and I asked: "Jim, when is the scope going to be in?" and he answered: "Lucille, it's already in. It's been in for some time." That's how good he was.

His success can be attributed to his amazing skills but also to the fact that he was a great communicator. I learned that he had minored in psychology, which is where I think he got his extraordinary listening skills. Jim knew how to put everyone at ease (except children). Kathy Yetman, his right hand staffer, was the one who got the children to stop crying. He had a warm, soothing voice and a soft chuckle with a wide smile when examining a patient. He was known to see some forty patients a day and never sounded rushed. He had a staff that was highly trained. His mind never stopped designing his next project.

Jim is still vivid in my mind. I particularly remember his last words as he was locking up his office door. The staff and I were already in the elevator holding the door open for him, but Jim was having trouble locking the door securely. Not wanting to hold us up, he called out: "I'm having trouble with the lock. You go on without me." Those last words have stuck with me as he did not return to his office again . . .

B. Raphael, PhD: There was flu going around New York and Dr Gould was so busy healing everybody else and, you know, "Physician heal thy self, it's nothing it's nothing." And by the time his wife Maureen got him to the emergency room they immediately admitted him and he died very shortly after that. It was something like double pneumonia that the flu had morphed into because he waited so long to treat himself, or to get treatment.

G. Korovin, MD: He had decided, right before he died, that he wanted to start slowing down a little bit patient-care-wise. So we were working on him cutting down to four days a week so that he could do research, and go to Denver, and be involved in other things. He was going back and forth to Denver. I used to look at him and wish I had the kind of energy he had. He would fly to Denver and back, go to work, but ultimately, to this day I don't know how he saw the forty patients and still got to the Carlyle at 4 am to meet with someone, which he used to do. Breakfast or tea at the Carlyle Hotel – I want you to join me with so-and-so at the Carlyle, and I'd think "How do you do all of this?" I still can't get out of the office until 7 at night! To this moment, I still haven't figured out how he did it, and I was there!

It seemed to come out of nowhere. We were doing an EPIC [Executive Performance In-Training Center] session in the office on the weekend, so I was with him all day Friday and Saturday. There were three people being trained, Lucille was there. To me he wasn't looking great, or strong, and then he was going to be interviewed on one of the TV channels about the Super Bowl the next day. He was preparing what he would potentially answer while other people were working with the people they were training. He had been given a list of potential questions, and one was about people having hoarseness after the Super Bowl. He had a percentage, and I said well, I don't know that I agree with that – my husband goes to Giants games, and I've gone, and three out of the four people in the car are hoarse when they leave, the one that wasn't was me, because I wasn't going to be an idiot yelling. So I said that to him that I thought the percentage may be higher.

The next day, there were two things about that show. I said to myself, he doesn't look good, he looks grey. I don't know if they had put makeup on him or anything, but there was this weird feeling I had. The other thing was that they interviewed him, and for one of the answers, he stated, "My young associate says that 75% of people who leave Giants games are hoarse." I said, "What did he say?" He actually quoted my number, using my name. There was no research, it was just a number! Later that day I called him and said, "You were great on TV," but I was worried. There was something that I just knew he didn't look good.

The next day he was too ill to come into the office. During the week, he called his cardiologist, and he didn't want to go in an ambulance, but the cardiologist went to his house, and went with him by cab to the emergency room at Lenox Hill. Apparently he was in ventricular tachycardia. They tried to convert him in the ER, and he ended up in ventricular defibrillation. They put him in ICU for a few days, and then he passed away. It was horrible.

It was daunting. It was literally overnight. I think he passed away on Friday, and I had to be there Monday to see patients. And now I had to tell all of these patients, who had come to see Dr Gould.

L. Carroll, CCC-SLP: Dr Gould had a lot of people (patients and friends) at the U.N., a lot of people in broadcasting as his patients. At Jim's memorial, held at the Ethical Cultural Society in NYC, there were three podiums where David Brinkley, Mike Wallace and Dan Rather stood and read one telegram after another. One was from President Clinton and one from Frank Sinatra, who had promised Gould that if Jim died before Frank, Frank would sing at Jim's funeral. Unfortunately he couldn't make it, but Bill Riley sang and Ben Vereen sang 'When the Saints Go Marching In', and there was this massive wreath of flowers and hearts that had been sent by *The Grateful Dead* (another of his clients).

The memorial started at 3 pm and went to 7 pm. At one point during the reading of the telegrams, Mike Wallace stood up and said, "It is five minutes to five, and your broadcast starts in four and a half minutes. We need to excuse Dan Rather." Who said, "Thank you very much" and quickly covered the block to his studio in record time.

R.T. Sataloff, MD, DMA, *1994 Gould obituary*: His contributions as an educator along with his devotion to his students, friends and patients, led him to be justly loved and respected as one of the truly great men not only in Otolaryngology, but in all of medicine. He will be deeply missed; but his values, traditions, curiosity, and insistence on excellence will continue on forever through those he trained, and those of us lucky enough to have been called his friends.

5

Ripple Effect

Almost anything in voice, if you scratch the surface hard enough and deep enough you'll find Jim somewhere.

J. Rubin, MD

Dr Gould mentored through example and inclusion, and the force of his entrepreneurial vision changed voice medicine and science. This chapter looks at some of the organizations that grew from, or were strongly influenced by, Dr Gould, Dr Sataloff and The Voice Foundation over the years.

R. J. Baken, PhD: Jim Gould was teaching a seminar at Columbia when I was a doctoral student. I was still not sure if I was going to focus on voice, but Jim made it clear that he thought I should, and he started to include me in all sorts of little activities, including work at his Vocal Dynamics Laboratory at Lenox Hill Hospital. Just after I finished my doctorate we co-taught a course. He continued the seminar, and I got added to it as a co-leader. Jim had a way of occasionally phoning me and others to say something like, "You will be at my office Thursday at 6 pm after I've seen my last patient. We have something to discuss." 'Something to discuss' meant we were going to sit in Jim's office and he was going to give us marching orders. Once he phoned me to tell me that I should go to a special meeting of laryngologists – at Jorge Perelló's office in Barcelona! It turns out that it was a very early meeting of the Collegium Medicorum Theatri. I've been involved with CoMeT ever since. Like I said: smart people didn't refuse Jim Gould.

L. Rubin, PhD: Jim invited me to observe his work with his patients. I jumped at his invitation and spent a few weeks watching him perform magic. This was prior to the advent of scoping, so getting to look down the same throat that Jim was examining was not easy; however, his assistant, Kathy Yetman, had me stand behind him while she pushed my head over Jim's shoulder so I could see what he was seeing – and I was thrilled. Throats of all sizes! Some opera singers had vocal space that seemed as large as a cow's throat! After my 'learning sessions' Jim would at times discuss the day over an ice cream soda next to his office or invite me to breakfast to discuss his next project. A few weeks after my time learning so much from Jim, The Voice Foundation became a reality. I signed up as a member from day one and have been an active member since then. Attending the 'Care and Training of the Professional

Voice' Symposia revolutionized my teaching.

A short time later, Jim wanted me on his premises to work with his patients, while I could also continue to coach my own clients there. He set me up in an office down the hall from his. I was lucky to work with so many of his patients who presented with unlike concerns. Having the back and forth communication with Jim was enormously helpful to me. He would send a patient to me and indicate what he wanted me to work on and how many sessions I should give that patient. After some time, I eventually found my own space as I needed a bigger room for my workshops, recording equipment and piano. But we still stayed in touch as Jim always had another project in mind. Those projects came to realization with EPIC and a multitude of workshops.

EPIC – Executive Performance In-Training Center, Ltd

From EPIC promotional literature: In a two-day total immersion program the EPIC team evaluates the participants' present vocal communication skills, helps them to identify goals and objectives and, through individualized intensive interaction sessions, helps them to begin to acquire those desired skills. A post-session training program is designed to maintain the realized skill levels. [...] Primary emphases are placed on imparting straightforward information, providing clear instruction, increasing self-awareness, and initiating a program of behavior modification. Although participants cannot expect to habituate these new skills in just one weekend, a solid foundation and methodology are laid out for ongoing developmental work.

L. Rubin, PhD: Jim's dream was to address the diverse needs of his patients and clients so he rented a space with many rooms, each attended by a trained coach. Those needs included: Relaxation, Throat Examination, Breathing, Singing, Public Speaking, Presentation, Vocal Therapy, TV Interviewing, and more as the need arose. That space didn't work out as he wanted, but his idea grew into EPIC.

EPIC sessions were long, intensive and held on weekends. Participants were frequently from a well-known corporation or firm with some four to six clients attending together. Weekend training started on a Friday night and ended late Sunday. John Haskell introduced the anatomy and physiology of the voice to the entire group by having them observe their throats with a light and mirror and by viewing a voice video. Then the participants went to separate rooms with a coach. Marie Torre interviewed and filmed each client for a TV experience. At the end of the training Marie played back the interviews for all clients to view. This helped them recognize how much they had accomplished (or hadn't).

Some of these training projects were held at Lenox Hill Hospital, some in East Hampton and others in Jim's office. (I remember working with Al Gore in Jim's office). Additionally, Jim wanted a handbook, Executive Training, made up to distribute to participants. I volunteered to put the book together with a chapter submitted from each coach, and I remember seeing a stack of them in Jim's office. As demand for the training grew, we began to offer workshops on various sites.

What I remember most from these experiences is that the clients were a joy to work with. Also, I believe Jim was indirectly saying to the participants that medical help is frequently needed for the distressed voice but patients and clients can also improve their vocal skills and avoid misuse and abuse by taking the training and doing the exercises.

At Gould's request I taught many workshops for traders on Wall Street to 'scream safely' in the ring (pit) and save their voices. One company overseer said to me, "Doctor Rubin, this guy is worth millions to me with his voice, but he's worth nothing to me without it." I got the message and at that time I was allowed an observation session in the ring (now defunct and replaced with modern technology). I had to hear the voices to know what traders were doing to their voices. Vocal volume was harder for the women to achieve because they did not know how to anchor their voices in their bodies. Most female traders used high frequencies and many, including the men were losing their voices. I taught Wall Street clients on my premises and on theirs.

B. Raphael, PhD: Dr Gould, through his office, put together a team of individuals. He was the head, and there was a speech pathologist, John Haskel, and I was there for the voice, from the theater field. Karen DeHio was a massage therapist who would help the clients relax and teach them exercises they could do when they were feeling particularly tense. Claire Alexander was the singing teacher and Marie Torre was the media specialist.

We met together on a Friday night and took a hired bus to the Hamptons. We started work right on the bus. We would talk, getting to know each other, talking about what our specialties were, getting to know the clients, asking him or her what the goals were. On Saturday we usually met as a group in the morning and had lunch, then the client or clients had individual sessions with several of us in the afternoon. Sometimes after dinner the client would deliver a speech so that we could see them in action and give them some coaching. Sunday was a similar schedule, returning to New York in the late afternoon. Between 1985 and 1994, I participated in around thirty sessions.

I taught them how to warm-up the voice and designed those warm-ups for their particular needs. So if they had an opportunity to warm up a little physically we did that. If they had to do closet warm-ups on the podium while they were being introduced, we did some exercises for that. And a lot of them had to loosen their ties if you know what I mean. They were uptight and powerful, authoritative, and consequently they were not very expressive facially or vocally. My job in particular was to work with them on greater spontaneity, and interview techniques like looking people in the eye, and answering the question without really answering it if you didn't want to, changing topic. Also, speaking more expressively in terms of pitch, instead of being monotonous, mixing it up a little to hold the interviewer's interest a little more. We all taught voice care: give up smoking, make sure you're hydrated, the usual stuff.

J.A. Haskell, CCC-SLP: Dr Gould liked to work with people. He was very interested in training, and had this idea of getting a small group of voice specialists together for an intensive weekend of training, working with accomplished speakers who needed healthier voices and could be even better speakers. He always felt that there was more to voice than being a doctor and doing what he did medically.

Dr Gould was interested in getting a staff of people who could get along, who could form a team. The original group had four training specialists. The acting-voice specialist was Bonnie Raphael, who is one of the top acting-voice coaches. The singing specialist was Claire Alexander, a voice teacher in New York whom Jim knew and had worked with. She had been an opera singer and in musical comedy. I was brought in as the speech pathologist, and the fourth specialist was Marie Torre, a newspaper writer and columnist, who was noted for her interviews. One of her claims to fame was that she had gone to jail for refusing to reveal sources for an article on Judy Garland.

There were a couple of other people who handled the technical part. The executive director was Gary Gatza, an attorney in NYC . . . a very nice fellow. EPIC was part of The Voice Foundation, sponsored by, connected to, TVF. It is part of the story.

In 1985, Jim set up three dates with the team going out to East Hampton. At first we stayed in the 1776 House hotel; then a year or two later he bought a house for this purpose. Gould already had his own house in the Hamptons and went out there frequently with his family. But he bought another house for this purpose where we settled in for these intensive weekends.

The first three intensive weekends were with an individual, to see how the plan worked, and how everyone worked together. Then, the following year there must have been four or five of these weekends with groups of three or four people. One of the people in the first year was Dan Rather. He was a patient of Gould's, and he was interested in this because he had developed voice problems during conventions and on election nights when he was on for hours. He was afraid that he would have the same kind of problems that his mentor, Walter Cronkite, had had. Cronkite had serious voice problems and had to have surgery. I don't know quite what the problem was, but Rather was afraid of that. When Jim mentioned this weekend, Rather jumped at it.

So, he was on the bus to East Hampton with a couple of people from CBS, very important people at CBS who were probably there to see that nothing happened to him. The weekend was very helpful for Dan Rather. One of the things we worked on was smiling. He couldn't smile easily. He was great at serious stuff, but he couldn't just relax and smile, in the way that Walter Cronkite could smile and make you feel good. So we worked on smiling. About six or eight months later, there was a cartoon in the New Yorker with a couple sitting on the couch watching television, and one of them says to the other, "Don't you think Dan Rather is looking a little more chipper these days?" Working with Dan Rather and so many other accomplished people, as well as with the other specialists, was one of the great learning experiences for me. We had wonderful weekends.

Then it broadened to not just the weekends. Jim and Gary set up special programs, all through EPIC, to go down to the NY Stock Exchange and do presentations for the people who worked there, yelling and screaming and losing their voices. So we did three different years of programs, an hour, hour and a half presentations, three of us doing things. Jim was interested in using this group in as many situations as he could. He actually took a group to help on the campaign trail in 1992. Gould had all these high-level patients, people he was working with, who needed work on their voices and presentation skills, their ability to interact.

We worked with a number of hot-shot lawyers, a number of people in government, two or three people from presidential cabinets. We did this until the weekend before Jim died in 1994. We did a one-day session in his office, with a congressman from Brooklyn. None of us knew that Jim was very sick at the time. That was the last one. The EPIC program was a great thing for all of us who participated.

Around 1990, he turned the project over to Bob Sataloff. Bob was interested, and brought his whole crew over to New York for a weekend out in East Hampton and they all went through the process.

R.T. Sataloff, MD, DMA: EPIC was a very good concept. The training takes a minimum of three ten-hour days. We did an intensive training on Friday, Saturday, and Sunday with one person and often 6-8 trainers. We had other models with more people for less intensive sessions, but we were always so busy taking care of patients and teaching, that we just never moved forward with it. But there is still a place, and if I ever get less busy, I would revive it.

Recording and Research Center for Denver Center for the Performing Arts

R.T. Sataloff, MD, DMA: It was Gould's idea. There was an opportunity to build a research center physically in conjunction with a recording studio and conservatory environment to train actors. Gordon Getty was interested in funding it. It was largely Gould's vision, done in collaboration with Ingo Titze and me, and largely with Getty's support. It has been a major center for research.

Unfortunately, the support was for the initial capital investment, and the Research Institute and

Recording and Research Center were not endowed. So, they have had to obtain their own funding in order to continue to succeed, but they've been generally successful in doing so. When Gould died, Ingo Titze essentially took over as the guiding scientific force in Denver, with ongoing collaboration and support from The Voice Foundation and from me.

I. Titze, PhD: Every year Gould came out to Denver for a few weeks. As a young physician, he had served in a military hospital in Denver, at Fitzsimmons Hospital. He asked me, would you like to run a voice laboratory out in Denver? I told him I didn't have the time, as I was already an associate professor at the University of Iowa. He said he wanted me there in whatever way it could be worked out, "Even if you come on as a consultant, and are only there for a day a week."

When Dr Gould died, the Denver Center for the Performing Arts changed the laboratory name from Recording and Research Center to Wilbur J. Gould Recording and Research Center. In 1996, when I received a large center grant from the National Center for Deafness and Other Communication Disorders, we changed the name once again, this time to the National Center for Voice and Speech because the large grant covered research at the Denver Center for the Performing Arts and three universities, Iowa, Wisconsin, and Utah.

B. Raphael, PhD: I distinctly remember going to the 1982 Juilliard Symposium and being interviewed by Dr Gould for the Denver job. My job at Denver was a split appointment; half my salary came from the Recording and Research Center and half my salary came from the theater company. So I was coaching the actors in the company and I was participating in research at the Recording and Research Center at the same time. That was really unique. It was pretty spectacular.

When he was interviewing me in the lobby at Juilliard, he was trying to run The Voice Foundation Symposium at the same time, and to spice that up a little bit, Dr Gould was treating one of a series of Broadway Annies in the lobby because that's the only way this little girl would get to see him, which was pretty typical of the way Jim Gould operated.

R.C. Scherer, PhD: I remember a conversation with Jim Gould at one of the Symposia because there was discussion of the creation of this new Recording and Research Center that Jim was going to head from New York. Ingo Titze was going to be the director of it, relative to the primary activities at the center. Jim Gould approached me and said, "Would you be interested in this position?" and I said, "Well, that's flattering, I'm not sure if I'm qualified for anything like that. Thank you very much for taking interest in me." He was almost insistent that I should consider the position. I'm thankful that he was, and it made sense at the time. Ingo wanted me to come out, and asked me to join them and that was wonderful so we all moved over to Denver.

I was the daily manager, the financial officer, a scientist, and an educator in the new Conservatory for training voice and speech coaches with Bonnie Raphael and the group. It was a great experience to do a little bit of everything, because I loved every minute of it and the variety of it.

But the financial underpinning of the research environment there at the Denver Center for the Performing Arts started to change over the years. We were needing to establish more federally funded grants and there came a time when that actually became quite difficult. I had always wanted to teach, and I also had a desire to return to Ohio where I grew up, so when the opportunity to go to Bowling Green State University came in 1996, I left the Denver Center for the Performing Arts. That was a good move for me because I really treasure teaching and promoting the research of students.

I've been extremely fortunate in my career to be associated with Jim Gould and Ingo Titze. It was extremely important to have both Jim and Ingo as my 'bosses' and that connection was very informative to me. These were very formative years for me. Jim was a visionary and leader with progressive ideas, as is Ingo. I owe a great deal to both of those gentlemen and learned a great deal from them.

W. Riley: The National Center for Voice and Speech (NCVS) started as the Denver Center for the Performing Arts (DCPA). The Symposium went to Denver in 1985 as an opportunity to showcase the Recording and Research Center at DCPA.

I. Titze, PhD: We are forming the Pan American Vocology Association, which is completely member-driven, reaching out north and south on the American Continents. One goal is to develop a level of certification for singing health specialists. The business part of the association is in place. A membership drive is ongoing. There are about fifty charter members. PAVA might be the continuation of the NCVS, and perhaps a partner with TVF.

About a year and a half ago, there was a meeting where we tried to find some consensus on voice teacher certification. We've debated terms like Singing Voice Specialist (I think that is a singing teacher) and Singing Health Specialist (which is more of a 'to be defined' specialty).

NIDCD – National Institute on Deafness and Other Communication Disorders

R.C. Scherer, PhD: The very important influence I thought that both Jim Gould and Ingo Titze had was developing the voice section at the National Institutes of Health (NIH). That was very important. Also, the function of The Voice Foundation and the Symposia was very important relative to the word 'voice' being separated from 'speech' so that people understood that the voice was its own entity to separate it out at the NIH.

R.T. Sataloff, MD, DMA: *Then the NIH started to separate out voice...*

That is correct. It used to be that neurology and otolaryngology were in the same National Institute. When otolaryngologic research was recognized as important, complex and multifaceted as it is, the National Institute on Deafness and Other Communication Disorders was formed. It was divided into six divisions. There were goals and objectives and research priorities that were set forth at the inception of the Institute. Gould was a representative to develop those materials for the Voice Institute, and we collaborated on them together. I actually wrote the draft of those criteria with him, and he had input from other people as well. So Gould and other active people in The Voice Foundation helped establish the research priorities that have driven the voice research component of the NIDCD.

L. Carroll, CCC-SLP: 1990 was the year of the first NIH meeting on voice in Bethesda. Dr Gould announced that Voice funding had reached the critical mass of 1% of the NIH budget. Minoru Hirano was there, Woody Starkweather and Katherine Harris were the US moderators, and Christy Ludlow was doing the work on spasmodic dysphonia. This was the beginning of the NIDCD.

Canadian Voice Care Foundation

K. Ardo: Dr Sataloff would say to me, "You have no idea how much you can do. You've only scratched the surface you just need confidence in yourself."

Dr Gould, oh my goodness, if it weren't for him, there wouldn't be a Canadian Voice Care Foundation, there wouldn't be my great interest in voice and in the health and vocal fitness of voice care. He was very much a part of that. That is why we have always put his name in the brochure for CVCF symposia.

I was one of the fledglings with Dr Gould for a while, going to New York several times from 1978 on. He would permit me to be in his office and to shadow him. Then I decided that Canada has to have a Canadian Voice Care Foundation so we can get together and make other people aware, and awaken this amazing knowledge for their use. It happened at a time in my life when because of the post-polio and my fears of tripping onstage, having nightmares about tripping onstage, it was a time to go into a different part of my vocal path. That path led me to The Voice Foundation, and to creating the Canadian Voice Care Foundation. I couldn't have done it without the support of Dr Gould and Dr Sataloff. Dr Sataloff would say to me, "You have no idea how much you can do. You've only scratched the surface; you just need confidence in yourself."

I went, I think, for twenty-eight years to the The Voice Foundation Symposia; participated, gave workshops, learned and grew. At one point, I think it was the year before Dr Gould passed away, we sat down together in the empty hall while I told him about my dream of having a world conference in voice care. Dr Gould and I talked about planning over five years, and taking the best of what had happened in five years and present it at a huge world conference. But that never came to pass.

After breaking both kneecaps recently, my travel has been limited. But I teach a lot, I give workshops, I do vocal fitness classes, and I try to pass on as much material that I've gathered in the last thirty-some odd years as I can.

Starting the Canadian Voice Care Foundation was a great learning experience. I'd never done anything like it before. I was helped by many people really, and knew that once the paper work was done, I would need somehow to do some fundraising. At the time, I was building up the voice department at the newly formed Red Deer College, which had just been built by Arthur Erickson, which is one of Canada's leading architects, and he had built this wonderful theater in Red Deer that really lent itself to have a meeting like The Voice Foundation does in the United States. And so, that's when it began to formulate in my head. We got the CVCF registered, a board, and then, in 1990, had the first big voice conference in Red Deer.

Red Deer is in the middle of nowhere. It's an hour and a half away from Calgary and an hour and a half away from Edmonton, the two major cities of Alberta. And we had close to three hundred people there from all over the world. Dr Sataloff, of course, was heading, and we based our format on The Voice Foundation, with one difference. Each presenter had half an hour to present with another fifteen minutes added for questions. It became a very thorough meeting where people really had the chance to take the time to understand what was being presented. They all loved it because they had more time to present and more time to say how they felt about things.

And we tried to have all three meals of the day together with the speakers at round tables which added to the camaraderie, the making of friendships and the understanding of the work that was being presented. It's wonderful to have founded the Canadian Voice Care Foundation and to have built all this understanding and passed all this wisdom on to people. On the other hand, to run such a foundation, with the cutbacks that we have had in the last twelve years made it very, very difficult.

Calgary's getting a magnificent new building, the Canadian National Music Centre to represent all of Canadian music, Canadian artists, and to have the

Juno nominations. We're hoping that the Canadian Voice Care Foundation will have a home there; that if I'm too tired to take it on, it will be carried on at the Canadian National Music Centre.

British Voice Association

J. Rubin, MD: The British Voice Association is in many ways comparable to The Voice Foundation, because it is multidiscipInary. It is very involved with the singing voice, the speaking voice, the pedagogy and clinical practice of voice. We have about 620 or 630 members at present. It's built on, I think, similar lines to The Voice Foundation. The people who were involved initially in the organization that ultimately formed the British Voice Foundation had spent time with Jim, and he certainly either directly or indirectly supported its development.

I'm sure it's a ripple of some sort. Almost anything in voice, if you scratch the surface hard enough and deep enough you'll find Jim somewhere.

The quantum leap, for laryngology was getting and learning to rely on the strobe rather than just using the flexible scope. Its use became the standard of care for the specialty voice clinic. Just looking with the naked eye through the flexible scope is still being used probably in most rural centers in America and many centers in the UK. The good news is that, and again I think Jim Gould had a lot to do with it, the British Voice Association now has over a hundred voice clinics registered with it throughout the United Kingdom. I like to think that each one of those voice clinics has a stroboscope and has at the very least a close working relationship between a surgeon and a speech therapist – that's really quite extraordinary.

Second World Voice Congress and Fifteen Symposia in Brazil

M. Behlau, PhD: Professor Sataloff improved my self-esteem a lot by coaching me, by helping me. And then the wonderful colleagues I have there always help me. It was a real partnership because they came here to give classes and take part in our national and international meetings. I started a specialization program in Brazil, working with the students to get specialized in voice, and every year I take students to the US. Those are Masters students, PhD students, or our first level of graduation before master that is the specialization – it is something similar to your CCC [Certificate of Clinical Competence]. These young students, they go, every year they present, they take part. In some years we have delegations with more than thirty Brazilians in the US. We are always the largest foreign representation there.

And I love the long hours, from 7 in the morning to 10 in the evening, I love it. I think this is absolutely great. I need to go and sit at the first row or the last to plug in the computer because I take notes and when I come back to Brazil we have something that is called 'The Feedback on The Voice Foundation' so I present to everybody that could not attend. We have a special meeting on what were the main issues at The Voice Foundation, and I have summaries like notebooks, small leaflets, for people with the ten best points of the Symposium each year.

Professor Sataloff invited me to join the reviewers of the *Journal of Voice* and I said, "Oh, I don't know how to do that." He said, "Yes, that's why I am inviting you. You are going to learn." So he started sending me papers and sending me the other colleagues' reviews for me to benchmark, to compare. Due to this process, I started writing better papers. So The Voice Foundation was a whole school for me.

I became an international member, then I became a professional member and I take part of the Board of Directors, Advisory Board, and *Journal of Voice* reviewers. Professor Sataloff improved my self-esteem a lot by coaching me, by helping me. And the wonderful colleagues I have there always help me.

Then I started inviting my American colleagues to come to Brazil. And we have organized fifteen symposia here in Brazil with the American colleagues such as Janina Casper, one of the founders of The Voice Foundation who was here, Lorraine Ramig, Kate Emerich, Daniel Boone, Joseph Stemple, Diane Bless, Nelson Roy, all these wonderful colleagues who came to Brazil.

We managed to organize the Second World Voice Congress and Professor Sataloff, himself, and all The Voice Foundation team were here. It was a real partnership because they came here to give classes and take part of our national and international meetings.

Center for Performing Arts Medicine at Methodist Hospital in Houston

C.R. Stasney, MD: We have great opera, symphony, and ballet in Houston, and since I've been the opera doctor for thirty years, I get all these calls from the symphony and ballet as well. So twenty-five years ago, I get a call from the symphony. They had a concert pianist with a problem with a thrombosed hemorrhoid who couldn't sit down, and they wanted to know if I could fix it. I said, "Well, I'm an ENT, but I know who could help."

Because of that, I started the Center for Performing Arts Medicine at Methodist Hospital in Houston. Now I have 164 doctors working for me and an endowed chair at Houston Methodist in Performing Arts Medicine. We take care of all the arts performers in Houston: symphony, ballet, opera and theatre, all the dance groups in Houston, as well as the Astros, the Dynamos, and the Texans. So whether they are big muscle athletes or small muscle athletes, we take care of all of them! I would love to take our model and expand it to every major city in the US so they all have a cadre of people in various cities to take care of performing artists.

Then Performing Arts Medical Association meetings got going during the summer in Aspen, and I was in charge of several of those. So I was conflicted between Philadelphia and Aspen – no offense, but Aspen won.

I believe in educating consumers, like on our website, TexasVoiceCenter.com, where I've put information I learned from Brodnitz and Sataloff. I tell everybody they are welcome to take it and print it. I got all this information from these great people, and I'm never going to have a copyright on excellence that I've borrowed from other people.

In 1994 I hosted, with Sataloff, a Voice Foundation First Annual Mini-Symposium. The faculty was Margaret Baroody, Marc Bouchayer from Lyon, France, Harvey Tucker, Austin King, von Leden, Sataloff and myself. It was an idea I had about taking TVF on the road.

The Contemporary Commercial Music Vocal Pedagogy Institute at Shenandoah Conservatory

J. LoVetri: The Institute exists as a separate entity within the university. We just finished our twelfth year in 2014. We have a three-part program that integrates a three-hour medical lecture based on Dr Sataloff's lectures at The Voice Foundation Symposia. I have attended his lecture for many years and I thought it was one of the most important parts of the Symposium. I still think so.

It seems to me a singing teacher needs to understand enough about voice medicine to listen to what an otolaryngologist or laryngologist is going to say about yourself or your students.

Additionally, Dr Wendy LeBorgne came to the Institute in year five to do a voice science segment in which she discusses formants and acoustics. She provides basic information so our participants can read and comprehend a voice science article. She also teaches a section on vocal health for those who complete the program as a bonus. Our medical lecturers there have been Dr Peak Woo, Dr Gwen

Korovin, Dr Michael Benninger, and Dr Chandra Ivey, and in 2015 we had Dr Adam Rubin from Detroit.

All three segments are taught at Shenandoah but I expanded the Level One trainings at the invitation of the University of Massachusetts Dartmouth, the University of Michigan Ann Arbor, the University of Central Oklahoma, and City College of New York. We have had Dr Norman Hogykian, Dr Scott Kessler, Dr James Burns, Dr Glendon Gardner, Dr Michael Pitmann, and Dr Perry Santos, as medical lecturers of those Level One trainings. All of them are laryngologists working with professional singers.

I also stress to our participants that even though you are taking a nine-day course you are not allowed to call yourself a singing voice specialist when you're done. We are not saying we make singing voice specialists. We are helping to create informed singing teachers.

I always bring The Voice Foundation information with me and always tell people my personal experience and suggest they come to the Symposia. I have invited many people into the Symposia, and a number of them are now talking about vocal health and vocal function in their own worlds and/or have presented research at the Symposia.

Growth of Interdisciplinary Team Work

J. A. Haskell, CCC-SLP: In New York, there are meetings of ENTs and SLPs four or five times a year, held at different medical centers, and the doctors there get together and talk about patients. Individual doctors present cases; sometimes the SLPs at an individual center present cases, so there is a lot of communication.

I coordinate a group of speech pathologists who specialize in voice (have done this for twenty years) and we meet four times a year, just to talk about professional things. There's a large group of people who come to these meetings. A lot of them are associated with hospitals, some of them work with show people and singers. We have pretty interesting discussions. In some sense it is an off-shoot of the Symposia and Gould.

There's a lot of interest in voice. The field has developed in all ways and it was inevitable that more and more people would be working in the area of voice. The field itself is much larger than when I went into voice. Lots of things brought this about. The Voice Foundation and the Symposia have done an awful lot.

It is all connected, and there is new ability to talk about things, new instrumentation. One of the exciting things a couple of years ago at the Symposium was a live medical session televised from Cleveland.

Back-Stories: *Katherine Ardo, C. Richard Stasney, Gwen Korovin, Ingo Titze, John Rubin*

Katherine Ardo

Singing Voice Care Specialist
Director: Canadian Voice Care Foundation

I had polio as a child, so as I was studying I always had to learn and feel my body and muscle memory as I was doing vocal production. This was especially true because I had a very big dramatic voice and often sang on raked stages. I sang in West Berlin for over ten years before returning to Montréal, and was always very interested in the voice, wherever I went. Even before Dr Sataloff and Dr Gould, I would seek out a laryngologist, so that they know what I looked like in my normal state and so that if I had something, they could see the difference. The interest was always there, even when I was very young.

C. Richard Stasney, MD, FACS

Otolaryngology
The Methodist Hospital, Houston
Elected Deputy Chief of Otolaryngology Service: The Methodist Hospital
Chairman: Center for Performing Arts Medicine, The Methodist Hospital
Director: Texas Voice Center
President: Texas Ear, Nose and Throat Consultants
Director: Van Lawrence Voice Institute at Baylor College of Medicine
Clinical Associate Professor: Baylor College of Medicine
Clinical Professor: Weill Medical College of Cornell University
Clinical Professor: University of Texas Medical School
Clinical Professor: Texas A&M College of Medicine
Adjunct Professor of Music: Rice University

What got me interested in voices in particular? The Houston Grand Opera. Van Lawrence was my predecessor, and one of the first laryngologists in the South. He, Gould and Hans von Leden were friends. They started Collegium Medicorum Theatri which is a group of folks from all over the world to take care of performers. Then Gould, Lawrence and von Leden started The Voice Foundation.

When I started my practice, I was doing a lot of cosmetic and ear surgery. But I was a back-up doctor for the Houston Grand just because I liked the opera. Dr Van Lawrence was the opera doctor and said, "Dick, you like the opera, can you cover for me while I'm out of town?" I didn't have a clue about voice care, and said, "What on earth do you do with opera singers?" He gave me a quick down-and-dirty course in laryngology, as there were no fellowships then.

Then Lawrence got sick with a melanoma, and as he got sicker and sicker, what was a tiny part of my practice became a major part of my practice, then when he ultimately died, I spent several weeks in Lyon, France with Marc Bouchayer, a very famous French laryngologist. His partner in Lyon, Guy Cornut, was a phoniatrician. Marc was the surgeon. My claim to fame was that I majored in French at Yale. Now they both speak English, but at that time neither did, so for a little window in time, I had a 'corner on the market' for laryngeal surgery in the South because I had learned from them and bought all of Marc's equipment.

So I spent time with Marc and I spent a lot of time in New York with Gould. There were no fellowships, so if you wanted to learn about laryngology, you'd go spend some time with Jim Gould or Friedrich Brodnitz and the folks that saw a lot of voice patients. I would watch Gould take care of patients, and be flabbergasted looking at the wall in his office. Everybody I'd ever heard of was on his wall. I loved going up there.

I became involved in the Symposia when they had just moved from Juilliard to the Manhattan School of Music in '88. I loved technology, and the strobes. That year I got the twelfth strobe unit in the US. There were many more in Europe at that time. Now Kay Pentax makes superb equipment, but my first were Brüel & Kjaer out of Denmark. For about twenty-five years I gave a two-hour course at the National Academy meetings on videostroboscopy.

I have enjoyed learning about the different aspects of the three professions that really deal with the professional voice, especially singers: the vocal pedagogues, speech pathologists, and physicians. We have emulated that down here, I have speech pathology and singing therapy readily available for all my patients. Frequently, I'll see a patient with a speech pathologist or singing therapist in the room. Sharon Radionoff works with many of the singers, and Steven King, the head of voice at Rice University, works closely with me as well.

Gwen S. Korovin, MD

Otolaryngology
Lenox Hill Hospital
Manhattan EET Hospital

If you were in a good Jewish family, you were either going to be a doctor, a lawyer or a teacher. I knew I wanted a career, I knew I wanted to support myself – it was one of those weird things, I didn't want to be reliant or dependent on some guy to support me. So I knew I wanted medicine or law. And I chose medicine because I like math and science. I went to stay with a cousin of mine whose husband was a doctor in the Boston area, and the night before my interview for medical school, he sat me down and asked, "Now, why do you want to go into medicine?" I gave him my reasons, and he said, "You know, all the women who were in my medical school class were really weird, so I don't know why you would want to choose that." And he is a psychiatrist. I don't think he should have been asking me that question when I'm there for a medical school interview. I thought it was the most bizarre question in the entire world.

I went to Cornell for undergrad. At Upstate I went through the medical school program. My father has a hearing loss. So my father said to me, "Hey why don't you take an elective in what's wrong with me?" That's a good idea, so I did, and took a two week ENT elective in the third year. One of the afternoons, they put us in a room where a woman was showing videos of vocal folds for the entire afternoon. That was Dr Janina Casper, who was involved with TVF from the beginning.

She showed videos of vocal folds, and there was something about that afternoon in 1983 that weirdly I would never forget. I sat there, and I was fascinated. Of all the different things, it was one of my most memorable afternoons, and at the time I didn't know why. I was fascinated by it, but didn't know I would choose ENT.

At New York Eye and Ear for my entire four years of the residency 1985–89, I was the only woman in the ENT program. I was only the third woman to ever go through the program. So it was an interesting period because of that.

So I had decided on ENT, and went to my first TVF meeting and saw Janina and thought, here is the woman who was showing those videos! And we became very good friends. She was an SLP, a research person, who did a lot of the first papers with Brewer and Woo. It was the G. Paul Moore lecture she gave one year. She was responsible for me being interested in laryngology.

I had to work at Lincoln Hospital in the South Bronx for three months each year, for three years in a row. Everyone was saying I would never live through it. Like I would literally never survive. The place was a horror show. The South Bronx was a war zone. The on-call room was in the basement, between nuclear medicine and the garbage. The room had panels missing in the ceiling and a bathroom with no hot water in it, and you would have to stay there an entire weekend. When I was going there, I got a key from somebody I had done my internship with who was also rotating through there on her surgical program, so I could get into the surgery on-call room on the fifth or sixth floor, to take a shower.

The South Bronx in the 1980s was an extremely scary place. It was unbelievable what came into the emergency room. There were bets in my program that I'd never live through it. You do what you have to do.

When I was finishing my residency, I was looking at what I wanted to do, what program, etc. Somebody said to me that Dr Gould, who I knew because I had been an intern and resident at Lenox Hill, was interested in bringing somebody into his office. The person who said it to me, was an ENT plastic surgeon, and he said, "I'll make a call for you and see if he's interested." He called me back, and said yes he is, call him. And very specifically, the message was call HIM and speak to HIM, versus contact his office staff. Talk to him on the phone, because no one else will know who you are.

And I did talk to him, and I remember saying something to my parents about it, and they said, "What, are you crazy? You'll never end up in a practice!" They thought I should go work for one of the managed care groups.

He said, "I'd love to meet with you, you can come in some afternoons and observe what is going on", to sort of shadow. But during the several months he invited me to do that, I was in the Lincoln Hospital rotation. So I would go from the South Bronx and go stand in his office and watch him. It was a bit of a contrast. How do you dress for that? Although I dressed better than most for Lincoln Hospital, it wasn't what you would wear for an upper East Side office. So there I was, he's seeing all these fancy patients, and I'm thinking "You wouldn't believe where I've just been . . ."

I would think, this is really crazy.

In the end, he said, "I'd really love for you to come practice with me." There had been a lot of just hanging out to see if I got along with his staff and everyone in the practice. It was extremely exciting for me; it was the dream to come out of residency into working with him. I was hired, but not full time, so to pay my bills I was also at the time working at a clinic down at New York Eye and Ear, and a clinic in Queens, I was all over the place. But then I would get this call from Kathy, Dr Gould's medical assistant and right hand forever, like a nurse practitioner would be today if they had the training, but she took all the calls, handled the big-time celebrities, and I'd be at my other work, one of the clinics, and she'd ask, "Dr Gould wants to know how long it will take you to get here" because he had somebody that he wanted me to be in on whatever it was.

The other jobs were paying the bills, but I wasn't really interested in them. So I'd get on the subway. So I was there more and more, and started to see patients on my own, and what started out being there a couple of afternoons a week, ended up growing into full-time. So I was kind of like a Fellow without being an official Fellow.

The second year I was there, in '91 or '92, he had a heart attack. He was told to stop operating, so he would schedule the surgeries and I would do them. The people knew, of course. He would come to the OR, and that was the best time for me to learn, because I would do the surgery and he would be there. It was like a Fellowship. Then he was cleared by the cardiologist to be able to go back to operating for a little while.

Gould's death seemed to come out of nowhere. We had just done an EPIC weekend in the office, and he had a Super Bowl television interview on Sunday. Lucille [Rubin] and I remember walking with him during the EPIC lunch break, it was really cold out, and he just had this little rain coat. We were walking and we were freezing, and she was on one side of him and I was on the other, walking with him, and she says she remembers him being really fragile and chilled, and asking him, "Why aren't you wearing a heavier coat?'

The next day he looked grey to me during the

Super Bowl television interview, and I was worried. At this time, Jack and I were planning our wedding, an informal, stand-around-the-fireplace ceremony on Mothers' Day. There were only a few people that I wanted to be there, and one was Dr Gould. I called him later that Sunday, told him our plans and wanted to make sure he was available. He said, "I wouldn't miss it for the world."

He was too ill to come in to the office the next day, during the week his cardiologist took him by cab to the emergency room at Lenox Hill. I remember getting the phone call. My phone rang, I guess it was a Friday night, and the phone rang really late, and nobody calls really late. So if somebody calls that late when you're home, you know it's either a wrong number or something really horrible has happened. I stayed up the whole night crying hysterically. It was just the most horrible thing that had ever happened to me. Thankfully, I had never lost a parent, but it was like losing a parent. It was everything. I felt close to him, he had really been helping, it was so wonderful working with him. I didn't know what the future was now, There was nothing set. It was a mess. And I was getting married three months later, and now when he had said to me, "I wouldn't miss it for the world." he wasn't going to be there. It was a really tough time, because I was also in the throes of keeping the practice going. We got married on Mothers' Day and took a very short honeymoon because I didn't want to be away that long. It was a crazy, terrible time; I was still depressed by him going.

So it was daunting. A lot of people didn't know what was going to happen. Eventually, it ended up that I bought the practice, and a lot of the people stayed with me. It was a crazy time.

I still think about him every single day. I really do. There is something that makes me think of him – like hearing his voice when I'm talking to a patient, hearing what he would have said. There are a lot of people who come in who knew him. Somebody usually brings up his name several times a week, actually.

Ingo R. Titze, PhD, MSEE

Executive Director: National Center for Voice and Speech, University of Utah, Salt Lake City
University of Iowa Foundation Distinguished Professor of Speech Science and Voice

I grew up in post-WW2 Germany, in Hirschberg, Silesia (an area between the Czech Republic, Poland, and Germany) when there was nothing much available for entertainment except the radio. My mother always wanted me to sing with her. She sang German Lieder, and we sang around the house and listened to opera. My father wanted me to study science. We emigrated when I was thirteen, and when I began school in the US, I kept the two areas of interest. When I was studying engineering and physics, I couldn't leave singing, and took lessons in my mid-twenties. My choice was to hang on to both the vocal arts and the sciences as long as I could.

While I was working as a research engineer for the Argonne National Laboratory in Idaho and for Boeing in Seattle, my mind was constantly on how the voice works, but I couldn't get answers. I would stand at the piano and wonder why I couldn't do what I heard other singers do.

While I was getting my PhD in Acoustics at Brigham Young University, I was introduced to Harvey Fletcher, the inventor of stereophonic sound, along with Bill Strong from MIT – they kept me going in physics, music, and speech. I still practice daily, do my vocal exercises and sing in concerts. I do one concert in the summer in Utah with vocology students, and one in winter at Iowa with acoustics students.

Early on, Dr Gould took me to some of his appointments, usually with politicians. We went to both Averell Harriman's and Ralph Becker's house to work with them vocally. I didn't contribute much – they were his clients – but hung around to see what prominent people are in need of vocally. He did this to teach someone in the vocal sciences, like me, how others could benefit from research. So I got a sense of how I, as a physicist, could affect people's lives.

Jim Gould was a person who could make himself small in front of large personalities. He got a lot of people to listen to him, and he listened very well himself. I learned that to be in the voice field you need to be very eclectic and interdisciplinary. I learned from him that you have to make the first step to approach people; they don't come to you. So I began to contact singing teachers, speech pathologists, and biologists.

John S. Rubin, MD, FACS, FRCS

Consultant ENT Surgeon and Lead Clinician of the Voice Disorders Unit: The Royal National Throat, Nose and Ear Hospital Division of The Royal Free NHS Trust
Consultant ENT Surgeon: St. Bartholomew's Hospital, London
Honorary Consultant ENT Surgeon: National Hospital for Neurology & Neurosurgery, University College London Hospital Trust
Honorary Senior Lecturer: Ear Institute, University College London
Chair: The Consultant Forum
Founding member: European Academy of Voice
Recent Past President: British Voice Association

There is no question that it was Jim Gould who pulled me into voice. What pulled me into being a doctor? That goes well into the dim and distant past. I think I knew I wanted to be a doctor when I was about six. At that time I think I wanted to be a plastic surgeon.

When I went through college I studied English Literature, and I spent a year at University College London as part of an exchange that Dartmouth College had at that time. I almost stayed on in English Literature, actually, but decided to continue on in medicine, so when I went back to Dartmouth I started the program and continued on to medical school in New York at New York Medical College.

I met Jim Gould back in 1979. That's a long time ago! I was a first year ENT resident and my chairman had organized a relationship between Manhattan Eye and Ear, which was the residency program I was in, and Lenox Hill Hospital, where Dr Gould was the head of the ENT department at that time. We each spent three months with Dr Gould at Lenox Hill Hospital, and I became very interested in the work he was doing. I actually walked across Central Park to The Voice Foundation Symposium that year. I didn't make it to the academic material but I got there in time to hear some of the Juilliard people singing which was really quite amazing. It was very different from the day-to-day ENT things that a resident got up to.

I kept in contact with Dr Gould as I continued through my ENT residency. That would take me through to 1981 when I did two years as a plastic surgery resident. I kept touch with him sort of at arm's length because I was very interested in his work but I didn't know for a fact that voice was going to be what I would end up doing for my life. In fact, I thought that I would probably end up as a head and neck reconstructive surgeon.

Then, after a head and neck fellowship as a lecturer for a year at University College London in 1983–84, I came back and touched base with Jim again. I became an assistant professor at the University of Maryland for a couple of years, mainly in head and neck cancer, but kept in touch with him and that's, I think, when I went to a Symposium again, after that brief vignette in 1979.

When I left Maryland, I went to the Albert Einstein College of Medicine in 1986, still ancient history, initially as an assistant professor. My chairman had a voice lab set up and left it under my purview amongst other things. So, I was doing head and neck cancer work but I was also doing some voice work.

In my voice lab, we had a stroboscope and I had a little camcorder that I had adapted and hooked up to a scope so we could take videos of people's larynxes. I had a very good relationship with a pulmonary physician as well as with a speech therapist. We developed a monthly interdisciplinary voice meeting at Montefiore where we'd sit down and look at interesting cases and talk about them and come up with medical, or surgical, or speech therapy treatment plans. It was a nice counterbalance to the head and neck work that I was mainly doing.

At the same time, I continued to keep in touch with Jim and to attend the Symposia, and ultimately I actually started working with Jim in his office on Wednesday afternoons in 1991. I got to know Linda Carroll, Bill Riley and Gwen Korovin who had also recently joined Jim in his practice; we had a lot of fun together. So I spent most of my time as a head and neck cancer specialist at Montefiore, and one session per week working with Jim in his office.

Jim had a number of big impacts on my life. As I said, if I had never met him I probably wouldn't have gone into voice. But there was more.

Jim was a sculptor, and one day when I was working with him on those Wednesday afternoons, at the end of clinic he took me along. That had a big impact on me. The people there were very interested in having another surgeon come and they got me involved. Sculpting and painting have become a very important part of my own life and that's again from having been encouraged by Jim to pick up a chisel.

Now I sculpt a little bit. It's very hard to find stone. Like Jim, I dislike using electric tools and chiseling stone can be tiring on the hands. Sculpting this way takes so long. I still have a couple pieces in my garden that aren't quite finished. I've also worked with wire and I've worked with clay. I mainly paint nowadays, with acrylics or watercolor. It's very intense, and extremely satisfying. I can't say I'm particularly good, but I find it very satisfying because when you get involved with something like that you just have to focus so much on it that you don't think about all your day-to-day cares.

6

Fiberoptics – Getting Behind the Curtain

> Looking at the throat through the nose with Gould's fiberoptic laryngoscope was novel, as you could look at the performer's throat without holding their tongue. That was a very big idea.
>
> P. Woo, MD

At the 2014 Symposium, groups of participants could be found during breaks, bobbing and weaving in front of well-lit mirrors trading advice on angles and fogging, using their slim smart-phones to photograph and video their own vocal folds as they spoke and sang. The curiosity, excitement, and wonder have not diminished in the hundred and sixty years since Manuel Garcia first watched his own glottis and larynx in 1854.

We know that earlier in the 1800s, physicians Garignard de la Tour and Philip von Bozzini used mouth mirrors for diagnoses, but vocal pedagogue, Garcia, gets the press because he was the first to figure out a way to view his own glottis out of a determination to better understand what was actually happening in there. The addition of fiberoptics to laryngoscopes, then the rapid evolution of stroboscopy as the fiberoptic light source became smaller and cooler, with the addition of increasingly high speeds of videostroboscopy, all opened new possibilities for voice medicine and voice science, expanding and increasing vocal technical understanding.

───────────

J. LoVetri: I'll never forget the first time I saw my vocal cords. I was scoped by Dr Stuart Selkin in the lobby at Juilliard, during a Symposium in the early 1980s. The monitor was where I could see it. I was just dumbstruck. "Whoa! There they are – my vocal folds!" I made every sound Dr Selkin requested because I could see how the folds were moving. I was just thrilled to see this. That was the first time I thought, "Oh my Gosh, when I think I'm doing so and so, I am doing so and so." What a revelation!

───────────

P. Woo, MD: Back in the 1970s, the instrumentation was fairly crude. The idea of being able to use a stroboscope to freeze motion, which meant being able to look at vocal fold vibration, was already known but it was always in the purview of a couple of laryngeal specialists, because there was no way to capture the information. But then, starting around the early 1980s, the first video machines came out, the beta max machines, and all of a sudden you didn't have to record this on a movie, but could record it onto a video machine. That was a terrific new idea. You could record the image and then play it back and analyze this image, instead of having to say, "Oh, this is what I saw" then quickly draw what you saw. So that was a very important possible research tool, even back then.

We've made some refinements to that machine so that today's machines are very versatile, to compare videos and do examinations. These were minor technical improvements, but in aggregate they helped people to systematically examine and re-examine what they were, and are looking at, and to be critical about what exactly they are seeing. It is fortunate that that all came about at the same time as the micro-computer, in the early 1980s. You could capture the image on a computer, and now we have people who capture the image on their iPhone. It is a confluence of technology and interest.

Looking at the throat through the nose, with Gould's fiberoptic laryngoscope, was novel as you could look at the performer's throat without holding their tongue. That was a very big idea.

The stroboscope had been around for over a hundred years. The electrical flash strobe was popularized by von Leden in the 1960s and then the newer things, the recording of the strobe was in the 1980s. It was not a single idea, but a conglomeration.

Now the computer cameras are much faster, so you can look at vocal fold vibration at a very fast rate. The vocal folds are vibrating at 100 to 1,000 or more times a second, so you need a very fast rate of capture to look at each individual vibration. So starting around the late 1980s, there was interest in high-speed, and before that it was all movie cameras, and Dr Gould did a lot of that work in the 1950s.

Dr Moore was the father of high-speed, with the movie cameras. Von Leden had a huge set-up at UCLA, and would make movie pictures of the throat at several thousand pictures per second. That was done only at UCLA. That's where Dr Moore did some of the work, and he also did some similar work at the University in Gainesville, Florida, all using cinematography. Then in the early 1990s, interest began in looking at the vocal folds with high-speed video. Now, it is possible to look at the vocal folds with high-speed video because of cheaper, better computers, and faster capture rates. Now, there are commercial systems that are available that can look at vocal fold vibration at thousands of times per second. Today, we use both the high-speed and the strobe to look at vocal fold vibration.

Videostroboscopy allowed people to have the visual aspect readily available rather than researching just the acoustic aspect. They used to have a lot of papers on the physiological aspects, filtering, electroglotography, things like that. Once it became possible to correlate that with the visual aspect, it became a new tool, adding the visual aspect at the same time.

———

In 1988, MIT professor Harold 'Doc' Edgerton was awarded the Presidential National Medal for Technology and Innovation for his innovations with the electronic stroboscopic flash. Along with the engineering and scientific sides of strobe lighting, the images Edgerton created are in museums, and his high speed stroboscopic short film, *Quicker'n a Wink* was awarded an Oscar in 1940. His wife, Esther May Garrett, was a singer and pianist and graduate of the New England Conservatory of Music.

———

R.T. Sataloff, MD, DMA: *Dr Gould's fiber-optic laryngoscope was presented as a new invention at the Sixth Symposium in 1977?* Correct. Machida company had just developed the fiber-optic laryngoscope, and the Symposia were among the earliest meetings in which its value for voice diagnosis was recognized. We began to develop protocols for how to use endoscopic information in a systematic way to understand voices and voice disorders.

At the 1980 Symposium, Dr Dale Tierney demonstrated a laryngeal fiberoptic stroboscope with videotapes? That's when we started getting enough low-light cameras and bright enough stroboscope lights to begin to be able to use stroboscopes in a practical way. It was really after 1980. It was closer to 1985 before things were really good enough to go into general use. But stroboscopy itself predated that 1980 presentation by a century.

Stroboscopes have been around since 1874, and people used stroboscopy to take care of voices beginning around the 1930s. The Timke stroboscope was bounced off doctors' head mirrors and used on a laryngeal mirror. It's just that the technology became good enough that it became practical to use and to advance in a scientific fashion.

Lots of us wrote and published papers on the value of stroboscopy. We had several of the major early papers on why to use stroboscopy, because initially there was resistance to it. People thought they were doing perfectly well without all the fancy equipment, and of course they were missing important diagnoses every day.

C.R. Stasney, MD: One of the problems early on, when people gave a talk about videostroboscopy, so much of the time they would talk about the lichen on the bark on a tree in the forest, and then you'd never know you were in the forest. The practical things that physicians ought to know they tended to miss, because there was this mystique about videostroboscopy, that made it seem so complicated that most people thought, "I'll never get that!" and it's not complicated. So when I gave my talks, I tried to make them as practical as possible, and to tell the physicians that unless I had access to videostroboscopy, I would never touch the larynx. It teaches you about the pathologies.

One of my first Fellows in laryngology, he was the finest resident to finish his program, and I told him, "Look with the mirror, make your diagnosis on a post-it and put it on the chart, then we will look together with stroboscopy." We would do that, and as bright as he was, and he was very bright, he missed the diagnosis 70% of the time.

So the technology really does help us. And it not only helps you make the diagnosis, but when you do a surgical procedure, unless you're stupid, you can figure out that *that* didn't work, and I'm not going to do it that way again. My favorite quotation from Ralph Waldo Emerson in 1841 is, "A foolish consistency is the hobgoblin of little minds." I love that quote, because so many physicians never get any better. You learn one way to do something, whether it's a rhinoplasty or operating on the larynx, and you do them all that way. And you may screw up every one of them. But you are just convinced that that is the way to do it. I think stroboscopy helps, because you learn that, "Hmmm, I got a lot of scar tissue doing it that way. Maybe I don't want to do it that way again."

H.M. Tucker, MD: Videostroboscopy has been extremely valuable to those of us who were interested in fine-tuning. It does give us some useful diagnostic information, but the main value of the videostrobe, to most of us, is documentation of the situation in the larynx before you do something to it. When I first started out, we did not have anything. We couldn't even take photographs. At the beginning you would watch someone's larynx with a mirror or with a right-angle telescope, and we would draw very careful pictures, on pre-printed forms so that they were uniform, of where a lesion was, what shape it was, what size it was, and how much of the larynx was involved. And then, you would write down your estimate of whether or not the vocal cord was limited in motion, or paralyzed, and so forth.

Video technology has allowed us to make very careful and very precise records of exactly what was seen before we do anything to these patients, which we can reproduce. We can use this to gauge whether or not we're getting improvement after things like speech therapy, for example. Where again, it's not only the sound of the voice that matters, it's whether or not things are moving the way they're supposed to.

Its biggest value to someone like me has been

documentation and results recording. To those of us working in professional voice it's even more valuable because you can pick up fine nuances of what's not working correctly that are not visible to the naked eye. You can slow it down so you can see individual vibrations and whether or not they're symmetrical, whether or not they are out of synchronization.

Videostroboscopy originated largely in Europe. Here in the United States, there was some early work in ultra high-speed, not video, but high-speed film which was at about the same time, but it had the disadvantage of being very expensive and very, very time consuming to get those records and then when video capability came into its own, obviously that's where we went.

There is a difference between high speed film and video. Video is not real. What you see. It is a continuous loop of images which appear to be what's going on, but in fact are just a sampling, a rigorous sampling. It gives the appearance to you as you look at it that it is ongoing, but in fact, only ultra high speed film can give you a real ongoing appearance of what is going on in the larynx. Suffice it to say, videostrobe, it gives you at least 95% of the information that you would get from the ultra high-speed camera and it's good enough, in most cases to answer the questions that we have. It has the one huge advantage that it has become relatively inexpensive over the years and it's available to any practitioner who does not need great technical skill once they buy a prepared unit that does all the work for you.

M. Benninger, MD: When I went to Detroit in July of 1988, we had the first strobe in Michigan and there had been none in Ohio when I left here. We got a B&K (Brüel & Kjaer), which was the standard stroboscopic machine, and then we got a secondary one up where I practiced out in the region, and that was a Nagashima, which had better optics than the B&K, but wasn't quite as popular, and subsequently went out of business. We started to do stroboscopies very early.

We pretty much looked at the larynx with a mirror the majority of the time when I was starting my training. By the time I finished, we were using flexible laryngoscopy and then we were going to rigid laryngoscopy and video recording.

The use of endoscopy or endoscopes has completely revolutionized our ability to better assess whatever organ we're looking at, and at the same time, do it in a less invasive way. If they couldn't see a patient's larynx well in the office, particularly before the late 1970s and early 1980s, they would put them to sleep and take them to the operating room to examine the patient under general anesthesia.

Easier office visualization of the larynx changed the whole approach to assessment. We expanded the use of these tools so that not only were we trying to make a diagnosis, but we were using these tools to be able to help us modify our therapies based on what we could visualize, see, hear or measure. The last thing it allowed us to do,was to truly validate our results because now we had some good subjective and very good objective tools, whereby we could say we've made this functional progress. It wasn't quite as anecdotal as it was before.

Things were a little anecdotal on treatment results, whether through non-surgical or surgical therapies, as it was not quite as clear as cancer therapy where you either cured them or you didn't. What we were looking at, were subtle changes in the voice support and sound. Patient perception about their voice quality and improved visualization of the vibration of the vocal folds allowed us to determine whether or not a lesion really played much of a role in the quality of their voices.

R. C. Scherer, PhD: When I was a student and in my early career, we had an old Wolf Strobe, but didn't use it much. We weren't in the clinical area at that time. I remember scoping myself all the time, though, and that was great fun and quite educational.

I remember when I was told that Minoru Hirano, back in the late 1970s, or so, was the primary person behind using stroboscopy on a routine basis in the clinic, whereas the rest of the world basically did not. He documented many cases, and through his work with Diane Bless and others, promoted the use of stroboscopy. Subsequently, it became state of the art. That is how I understand the history, but of course I could be wrong.

What I would like to see now, is that these more high-speed video instruments become the state of the art in the clinical world. I would say that the science of voice has moved forward because of greater resolution in time, greater resolution in space (whether that space is outside the tissue or inside the tissue), and greater precision in surgical procedures. Those are great advancements, plus the improved training of practitioners in the various disciplines of voice.

Stroboscopy and videostrobe technology were more established in European and Asian voice labs and medical offices before they caught hold in the United States. The question was asked, "Do you have a theory as to why this was so?" Here are several responses:

I. Titze, PhD: Optics has been the number one technical development in Germany. Optical instrumentation was the territory of Germany, so there has always been more instrumentation available.

But in the 1970s and 1980s, the research on videoendoscopy of the larynx was primarily in Japan, the US and Scandinavia. In the last decades it has been growing in Central Europe, specifically in France and Germany.

P. Woo, MD: In Europe they have phoniatry, which is a branch of medical speech pathology, so they had different types of specialists. Whereas, here in the United States, we had more laryngeal specialists that dealt more with cancer. Maybe the interest in vocal fold vibration was not as great in the United States.

There weren't more than a hundred stroboscopes in the US in 1980. There weren't a lot of papers presented at laryngeal meetings about vocal fold vibrations, or voice. Once people got used to the idea that they could show a visual image, it became more widely used in presentations, and certainly at The Voice Foundation the videos became more and more popular.

K. Ardo: The different provincial health plans didn't recognize using the stroboscope. It was very slow coming to Canada. The instrumentation in West Berlin when I was there was very much further ahead than it was here in Canada. If you went to an otolaryngologist in the 1970s, you'd have the little heated candle that would take Garcia's mirror and heat up the mirror and be able to visualize the vocal folds. That started to grow quickly and exponentially in the late 1970s and 1980s. But even today, otolaryngologists in Canada that have all of the equipment for the strobo-videolaryngoscopy are few and far between. Unless you have a voice clinic, they might have the scope, but they would be using it just as a scope; not everybody is set up for all of the acoustical or the visual equipment.

My background is Hungarian. So, in Hungary, Austria, Czechoslovakia, Yugoslavia, Russia, all of these countries, if you wanted to study and become a professional person, a medical person, a teacher, any kind of a profession, you had to be able to be fluent in German because the books were written in German. And I think from there, it evolved. Surgical equipment was made in Germany and Austria and they evolved as the centers of learning. Thus, the Germans were ahead in medical studies, building of medical tools, building medical surgical equipment, all of the things that have evolved. There was a great surge in Europe, in Germany, even before the wars. This is how I perceive it anyway.

M. Behlau, PhD: There were some strobes in Brazil and, soon after the first American or German strobes, they launched the Brazilian strobe: Unity. In the 1980s, at my university, we were actually the first teamwork effort in doing strobes and analyzing vocal fold behavior via stroboscopy. So we were one of the first groups working with that.

C. Sapienza, PhD: A theory might be the way in which the programs in Europe were funded. They had more government funding, or what you would call 'state funding', and they were selecting premier programs in Europe to be branded as the top speech science and audiology programs.

It always seemed like Sweden and Copenhagen, and different places were ahead of us. I think they were a little bit more prolific than we were, and possibly wrote about it more. They were doing kymography, which really wasn't necessarily that much more sophisticated, but it appeared to be when they presented it.

R.T. Sataloff, MD, DMA: By the mid to latter 1980s there probably were a hundred video stroboscopes in the United States. The Europeans had used the Timke stroboscope, bouncing it off their head mirrors, more than we had in the United States. So when the video stroboscopes became available, Europeans and Japanese doctors were already using stroboscopy, and they advanced the clinical application a little more quickly than many US otolaryngologists. It wasn't going from no strobe, to strobe; it was going from a mediocre strobe, to a better strobe.

The better early modern stroboscopes were made in Europe. The first by Wolf in Germany, and then by Brüel and Kjaer in Denmark; and it was the Brüel and Kjaer strobe, with a new light source developed by a fellow named Hans Peter Olefson, that really was the first one that was good enough for high-level video stroboscopy in routine clinical use.

I think that I had my first Brüel and Kjaer stroboscope in around 1985. I'm guessing on that. I still have four of them sitting under a desk in the office.

7

The Art of Laryngology ~

In medicine, you have to remember the milk of human kindness and how important humanism is in medicine. How important the holistic care of patients is.

F. Brodnitz, MD

H. M. Tucker, MD: ENT may appear to be a subspecialty, but it is really a very, very broad discipline. Sixty percent of all chief complaints are in the head and neck, and except for neurosurgery, we take care of all of them. Laryngology is also much broader than it would appear, even though it is a limitation by anatomic area.

G. Korovin, MD: One of the things I learned from Dr Gould is to really listen to the patient. People talk about that a lot more now, but previously it was "I'm the doctor, you're the patient, just listen to what I have to say." But if you really listen, most of the time they will give you the diagnosis, and you don't have to figure it out. It is within what they tell you. He was amazing that way. Really getting a full history, and getting a very extensive head and neck exam. Really checking everything, because someone may just have a blocked ear, and that's what's wrong with their voice. Everybody always felt that they were really listened to and taken care of, even if he was in there for a very short period of time.

It sounds strange to us now, because it's talked about at all the meetings, but people didn't do that. I still have patients who come in and say they went to the doctor and said they have a problem with the ear, and the doctor only looked at the one ear, not even looking in the other ear. Excuse me? It is the most bizarre thing, but this still goes on.

He had this whole thing about three deep breaths. He was always teaching people that if they were going to give a speech, to take three deep breaths before you say anything.

I actually said this at his memorial service; that I always felt that he had a sixth sense, because sometimes someone would come in with something that you would think was relatively nothing or minor, and he would say, "Well this is going to go this way", indicating that something was going to go bad, or a problem was going to occur. I wondered, "How did you know that?" Sure enough, a good portion of the time, it would go that way. It is true that he trained in a different time than now, where he didn't have all the tests that we have, so they really learned physical diagnosis better, probably, than the doctors of today. He always had that sense. We practice defensive medicine now, which he didn't have to do.

C.R. Stasney, MD: Gould was a genius. When Van Lawrence got involved with taking care of the visiting opera singers for Houston Grand Opera, he treated the first four or five bass-baritones for laryngitis. Later, he was having dinner with Gould in New York and said, "We've had a rash of red larynxes in bass-baritones." Jim said, "They all look like that, that's the way they are, they're not sick. In the words of Punt, a very famous English laryngologist, 'Bass-baritone vocal folds look like rose-colored satin slippers.'" Punt's daughter was a coloratura opera singer.

G. Korovin, MD: Elite singers helped create laryngologists. I think that opera singers notice the slightest changes in their voice.

M Hawkshaw, CORLN: I appreciated the need to develop the field of laryngology. When I started with Dr Sataloff there were three laryngologists' offices in the country where you could get strobovideolaryngoscopy, or that had a voice center. And it was Dr Gould's office, Dr von Leden in Los Angeles, and our office. And now, as you know, there's multiple voice centers in every city, every state, every country, and that's been hugely satisfying.

Laryngology just grew in leaps and bounds. Every fall, there's the American Academy of Otolaryngology, Head and Neck Surgery meeting, and we used to teach a strobe course on the heels of that meeting. We used to teach a three-day strobe courses at various places around the United States. Dr Dave Brewer was very active also, in the early years of our annual Symposium on Care of the Professional Voice. There was a lot of resistance, people raising their eyebrows, to bringing the three disciplines together: speech, singing, and laryngology. It was not an easy task!

J. Rubin, MD: For laryngologists, advancements in technology have revolutionized everything we do.

One example is the laser. We were very early users of the laser at the Royal National Throat Nose and Ear Hospital. I think we were the earliest users of the laser in the UK for voice issues. One of my colleagues, David Howard, was a forerunner in the UK in use of the Laser for Laryngeal Cancer, starting to use it in the 1980s. It was a natural development that it be used often in his, and later my practice of laryngology. Thus, all of us working there began to use the laser in clinical practice on the larynx.

The stroboscope is probably the single piece of equipment that most revolutionized what we do because it allows us, albeit not in true slow motion but in apparent slow motion, to visualize the vocal folds. And that's made such a difference because all of a sudden you have a very good idea as to what the viscoelastic properties of the vocal folds are. It is the viscoelastic properties that are critical. I think that's something that became very clear to Jim very early on.

Jim was very active in some of the early stroboscopy work and high-speed photography work. I think if you look at his 'bib' you'll find some articles with him doing high-speed photography which effectively look at the vocal folds in true slow motion, from probably the 1970s. As I said, everywhere you look you'll find his fingerprints.

But it was the stroboscope that was crucial from a clinical perspective. There are other modalities that allow you to see in slow motion, but the stroboscope is still the clinical tool that we use most often in the clinic, now often augmented through distal chip-tip technology and high definition technology. It allows us to improve in the outpatient clinic on our assessment of vocal fold function, in particular on the vibratory characteristics of the vocal fold and the likely causes of the vocal problem, be they due to scar or stiffness. The vocal folds may look absolutely perfect to the unaided eye, and yet they may have a very disordered function, and the crucial thing is function. And again, it was Jim who led the way on that.

M. Benninger, MD: The problem that I have from a clinical perspective, and particularly a physician clinical perspective, is that healthcare financing and healthcare economics are forcing us to really restrict our time with patients. Because of that, I don't think our current audio measures of voice are very helpful in the clinical setting, because we don't have time to do them or analyze them. High speed imaging for example is great, and we have high speed video imaging in our clinic but we use it primarily for research since we don't have time to do it routinely in the clinic.

Despite the fact that I think there are real opportunities to better determine whether or not certain measurable parameters, like jitter and shimmer and those kind of things, have any validity in helping us assess patients, I think the real challenge going forward is creating a short battery of tools that are reliable in evaluating any patient with any voice disorder and having that be done quickly enough that we can do it in the clinical setting

We don't currently have that. We have stroboscopy, which gives a very good, quick impression of what's going on with vocal fold motion and vibration and how it may affect a person's voice. Some other things are quick and reliable, depending on the patient: airflow analysis, or maximum phonatory time in vocal fold paralysis patients are good. I think our quality of life instruments like the Voice Handicap Index (VHI) are very good and give a relatively rapid assessment of the impact to the patient. And now we have the VHI for singers and the VHI for kids. We have other tools that measure quality of life, and I feel that there is almost no way to figure out what you should do with somebody before you see them. You have to establish a process where you can get that information quickly without disrupting the flow of the clinic.

In my practice, we use an electronic tablet that is given to the patients as soon as they check in at the front desk, so that we have that data available for us when we see them. It is challenging in that some patients have multiple complaints and trying to get them the right instruments may be difficult.

For example the patient may really be there for cough and not there for voice, or they are really there because of reflux and they are not there for either cough or voice, or the patient is a singer so they should get the singing VHI rather than the speaking VHI. So I think those tools are pretty good in the office setting, but we need a battery of three or four things that we can do as a global assessment of any patient with a voice disorder.

The other innovation from a clinical standpoint, is office-based procedures. On any clinic day I do three or four office-based procedures which were things that we would have never done before: injections and lasers, and those kind of things. I think that the future in that specialty would be better injectables, and even better laser refinement to be able to do more in the office. These are both time and cost efficient.

G. Korovin, MD: The other thing that Dr Gould was great at, was adjusting his personality – he was almost a chameleon. He was able to deal with all these different performers on different levels. You would almost see him change. Not his personality, but the way he related to these people. That was another interesting thing, how he related to them, even though they might be fifty years younger than he was. He was great at it.

A lot of it sounds kind of obvious now, because we have more people that practice like that. But at the time, that was very unusual. They would go in with whatever their problem was, like their nose was messed up from drugs, and he would never be judgmental about it, he would just take care of them. Let's just deal with what's going on right now.

All those patients, he was able to deal with them all. I learned that from him,

---

C. R. Stasney, MD: I was giving a talk on the videostroboscope at the Manhattan School of Music, and Friedrick Brodnitz, he was a great gentleman, a sweetheart of a guy, was there. I was talking about all this great technology and how we could tell if a gnat was circumcised with this technology, and he said, "Dick you may have great equipment, and I don't disagree with that, but in medicine you have to remember the milk of human kindness, and how important humanism is in medicine. How important the holistic care of patients is."

I have always tried to live up to that, so my patients know that I really do care for them and try to do for them what I would do for my own family, should my family be in that situation.

G. Korovin, MD: It is gratifying to take care of performers – to know that you are doing something to help people, and that you are able to get somebody back performing, or on stage because of something you've done to help them. It is gratifying and rewarding. And I love to go hear them perform and know that you've had a hand in that.

I learned to listen from Dr Gould, and I think some of it was also innate, because what I actually love about what I'm doing is the fact that, even though I never wanted to become a psychiatrist, there is a lot of that. A lot of it is figuring out the right approach to somebody.

I really care about what happens to these people, and I spend a lot of time. I enjoy listening to people, and I like to know, from a medical point of view, what is going on in their lives. I'm not gossiping, it is related to what's going on for them. People never really volunteer all the information at first, it happens as the exam goes on. The more time you spend with them, and we don't have all the time in the world, but the more time you spend with them, the more you find out what is helpful to what is wrong with them.

In November 2014, Dr Sataloff was the guest speaker for the National Association of Teachers of Singing monthly on-line webinar, NATS CHAT, bringing his trademark clarity and insight to a wide range of questions from the participating voice teachers. His answers combined the precise knowledge of a top otolaryngologist and master educator, with the experience gained from being a voice teacher and having been a performer and choir director himself (one of his students had just been tendered an invitation for an audition at the MET).

The questions came from issues that appear regularly in vocal studios and around which there has been conflicting information over the past decades: vocal fry, snoring, asthma inhalers and vocal atrophy, PMS and diuretics, over-the-counter medications and oral birth control, the effects of hormone levels on the voice through the stages of menopause, muscle tension dysphonia, and finally, respiration techniques and voce di sprega. This last was from another laryngologist, and the following is a partial quotation from his answer addressing the possible deleterious effects of belting (Dr Sataloff's full answer can be found elsewhere in this book in the chapter 'In the Trenches').

R. T. Sataloff, MD, DMA: There are lots of misconceptions about belting. The first thing someone needs to understand about belting, no matter what other technical approaches one wants to take, is that great belters are not shouters. Whether we are talking about the current high-belt trend in adults, or whether we are talking about these poor eight to eleven year-olds trying to sing Annie, if you listen to the ones who end up in our offices, they have a fairly constant volume with little change in vocal output, and are essentially shouting.

If you listen to, and study a great belter you will have trouble finding a single note that is the same from beginning to end. [The] variation, note by note, whether it is volume, vibrato, pitch, or all of them, is infinite. […] If they do it loud all the time, then they are going to end up in your office or mine.

Dr Sataloff's practice directly reflects his adherence to, and belief in the principles underlying The Voice Foundation. In the words of Margaret 'Peggy' Baroody who has been a part of the Sataloff voice team since 1991, "Bob believes that voice therapy and habilitation should be tried by all patients, singers and non-singers alike, before surgical intervention is pursued (except in very rare cases). This is the highest standard of care and he has never wavered from it, even though for a private practice, this extensive therapy protocol does not necessarily prove financially advantageous. That is literally putting your money where your mouth is!"

Peggy is currently one of the leading experts in the field of clinical singing and voice habilitation. She was a patient of Dr Sataloff while pursuing a performance career.

M. Baroody: I had also taught voice since my early twenties and in my mid-thirties decided to make teaching my primary focus. I had always had an interest in vocal anatomy, physiology and vocal pathology. When I asked Bob how to further my knowledge, he suggested that I attend the Symposium, at that time still in New York, which I did. While I did not understand half of what I heard that first time, I was hooked! I went back and spent more time with Bob and his team, who kindly shared their hard-won knowledge with me. Bob began to refer some patients to me. About a year or so later, he called me out of the blue to offer me a full-time position with his practice. I felt that this was an opportunity meant to be and I have never really looked back. I am more grateful than I can ever express to Bob for giving me this opportunity and making my education in this field possible.

As the senior voice clinician, my main responsibility is to make sure that as a team, the voice clinicians are functioning according to Bob's paradigm for care of an injured voice. That model has evolved over the years, in response to the natural evolution of the needs of our office, our patients, and best-practice concepts. However, the basics of patient care have remained the same. In the twenty-three years that I have been with this practice, many speech pathologists and singing voice specialists have spent time in our employ, only to go on to other practices when the time was right for them. I think that we work as a true collaborate team and I am proud to be a member.

8 ~ A Surgical Specialty

Dr Hirano's research on the layered structure of the vocal fold was revolutionary, as well as Dr Gray's basement membrane research. That was really groundbreaking...the laryngeal and phonosurgeries have really changed based on a lot of the research from our scientists.

M. Hawkshaw, CORLN

P. Woo, MD: I chose being an ENT because it is a surgical specialty, so you can help people fairly quickly, not dealing with chronic illness so much. When you do surgery on polyps, they would have a good voice within a week.

R. T. Sataloff, MD, DMA: When I first trained, there were just big ugly cup forceps, and laryngeal surgery was involved mostly with grossly stripping the cover off the vocal fold. As we came to understand the complexity and delicacy of the anatomy, people began designing much more precise instruments. Marc Bouchayer in Lyon, Robert Ossoff in Nashville, myself in Philadelphia, and others designed very delicate precision instruments that allowed much more accurate surgery, and resulted in better outcomes. Those instruments also allowed us to develop much more sophisticated surgical procedures, and those instruments have remained popular and relatively unchanged. There are now about a hundred Sataloff instruments available.

Bouchayer instruments, some of the Ossoff instruments, and later instruments by Mike Benninger all have enhanced the delicacy and precision of microscopic laryngeal surgery. Interestingly, the two of us who designed most of the instruments, Mark Boucher and myself, both were neurotologists, and much of our laryngeal instrument design carried over from our training and skills as ear micro surgeons and ear-brain interface surgeons. We used otologic precision surgical knowledge and transitioned it to laryngeal surgery.

As an anecdote, Marc and I knew each other for years through The Voice Foundation as laryngeal surgeons, but I didn't know that he was a neurotologist and he didn't know I was a neurotologist until we ran into each other at a neurotology meeting in Europe. We just looked at each other across the room and started laughing. It made perfect sense to us from what he had designed and what I had designed that both of us did so because we were ear surgeons.

M. Hawkshaw, CORLN: Laryngology is a subspecialty of otorhinolaryngology–head and neck surgery. A lot of doctors specialize either in otology, rhinology (diseases of the nose and sinuses), or laryngology (voice, and anything related to the vocal folds). There are overlaps with everything, including head and neck cancers, which overlaps with laryngology. Bob's practice has been limited to neurotology, which is ear-brain interface. He did a fellowship in neurotology. That means he can do skull base surgery. He can enter the brain – acoustic neuromas, big tumors, you know, and the skull base, not every ear doctor does that, you need to do a fellowship in that.

The laryngology fellowships started more than a decade ago. There used to be only six fellowship programs, now there's probably more than fifteen. Now, all the applicants that select laryngology go into the Match® program, and then we have to wait and see who they match us with. So it's good and it's bad. There's a ton of good applicants and the positions are limited. Before, we used to know our fellows one to three years in advance, because you could pick and choose. Now we don't know who we are getting next year until we see what the Match® turns up.

Everything you read will tell you that the flexible nasopharyngeal laryngoscope revolutionized laryngology. Everything changed after that, as did stroboscopy, when we were able to look at the vocal folds under slow motion, or at least cycles of vibration. Dr Hirano's research on the layered structure of the vocal fold was revolutionary, as well as Dr Steve Gray's basement membrane research. That was really groundbreaking. Botox® was a big change and changed a lot of treatment. And then we can't forget reflux. But I think stroboscopy has been the biggest advancement in voice care.

The tools keep evolving and surgical techniques keep changing, although analysis and evaluation are pretty much the same. In terms of video stroboscopy and nasopharyngeal laryngoscopy the tools are the same, but the surgeries have really changed, based on a lot of the research from our scientists, starting with Hirano and Gray. The laser is not popular with every laryngeal surgeon. Medialization and injection laryngoplasty continue to change. In the 1980s, everybody was injecting Teflon, but it caused many problems such as granulomata. We now use autologous fat, Gore-Tex® and Silastic®, Radiesse® voice gels. Things like that.

H.M. Tucker, MD: At the end of my year internship, I had applied for a residency in ENT at Jefferson in Philadelphia. My professor was a retired Navy double ENT, what we would now call an Otologist, or an ear specialist. Everyone else in the department had been protégés of Chevalier Jackson, the father of modern otolaryngology. They concentrated on doing rigid endoscopy, invented by Chevalier Jackson: rigid endoscope, rigid esophoscope, and rigid laryngoscope. In those days, most of what we now refer to as head and neck surgery was done by general surgeons or plastic surgeons. At the time that I was in training, this was changing to what is true now, where the vast majority of this is done by otolaryngologically trained people.

I was more interested in the neck part, the larynx part, than I was in the ear, although I had to qualify in ear. I ended up taking a fellowship concentrating in laryngeal surgery for cancer in which we were working on how to preserve the larynx rather than having to do a total laryngectomy.

While I was there, I was required to do a research process, and had read a paper about somebody who was talking about reinnervating the larynx. At the time, the interest was whether or not we would ever be able to transplant a human larynx and if you were going to transplant a larynx, there had to be a way to make it work. Unlike a heart where you can take it, and put it in and it will work, or a kidney, and it will work, a larynx will require innervation and muscle action to make it work. The larynx is the crossroads between your swallowing and your breathing . . . it's very, very important that it will work correctly or you will die of aspiration pneumonia.

I devised a slight improvement on how to go about getting the larynx to work after it had been transplanted and my triologic thesis was in reinnervation of reimplanted canine larynges. This technique could be worked over to take care of vocal cord paralysis which is a big problem in voice and it occurs fairly frequently. And, to make a very long and involved story short, I was able to develop a way to use these reinnervation techniques for the larynx to manage people with either bilateral or unilateral vocal fold paralysis and that is how I got in to voice.

M. Benninger, MD: From a physician and surgeon's perspective, I would like to study how to reduce scar. How to do surgical procedures in the larynx where we can be pretty sure that the normal vibratory vocal fold function would recover without scar or stiffness. The value of that would not only be with the obvious voice disorders such as resecting vocal masses from the vocal folds, but would be dramatic in patients with more complex problems, such as stenosis or webs, where when you open them back up they tend to re-scar.

People that have had vocal fold scar are very difficult to get back to a completely normal voice. I think from my perspective that would be the thing that I would like to really see from a research standpoint: reduction of scar.

There are thousands of unanswered questions:
- In vocal fold paralysis, does reinnervation really make much difference?
- Do different size prostheses impact medialization?
- Do we really need to rotate the arytenoid in vocal fold paralysis?
- For nodules, polyps, and cysts, do we really need to do a microflap?
- What are the roles of lasers?

It would almost be impossible to answer the ones that are the highest priorities unless you know which of the specific areas and disorders are to be addressed.

Back-Stories: *Robert T. Sataloff, Linda M. Carroll, William Riley, Mary Hawkshaw*

Robert Thayer Sataloff, DMA, MD, FACS

Otolaryngology, Otology, Neurotology, Skull Base Surgery
Hahnemann University Hospital
Thomas Jefferson University Hospital
St. Christopher's Hospital for Children
Department Chair, Professor for the Department of Otolaryngology-Head and Neck Surgery, and Senior Associate Dean for Clinical Academic Specialties: Drexel University College of Medicine
Adjunct Professor, Department of Otolaryngology–Head and Neck Surgery: Thomas Jefferson University
Adjunct Professor, Department of Otolaryngology–Head and Neck Surgery: University of Pennsylvania
Adjunct Clinical Professor, Department of Otolaryngology–Head and Neck Surgery: Temple University
Faculty: Academy of Vocal Arts, Philadelphia

When I was a child, I hadn't planned on singing, and didn't start singing until I was about thirteen, but I'd been planning on being a physician since I was about two. Since I was thirteen, I have mixed music and medicine. My voice changed when I was eleven, and it was much lower than it is now – we thought I was going to be a Russian bass – and I loved singing. So, I started taking lessons and gradually my voice matured into being a baritone like everybody else's.

My family heritage is Russian, I collect Faberge enamels and jewelry, it is sort of in the blood. I studied Russian music with Alfred Swan, an extraordinary Anglo-Russian who grew up in Russia, studied with Mettner and Scriabin, and his class left me with a lifelong passion for Russian music. He also gave me copies of Russian art songs, much of it by Balakirev, much of it [set] to poetry by Lermontov, which was pretty much destroyed when the publisher was bombed in the war. But it is extraordinary art song, as least as good as anything by Schubert, Wolf and Fauré. So I couldn't resist the opportunity to sing that from time to time so people could hear it, because it's never been republished. My DMA dissertation was in three parts: a paper on Music Health and Performance, a recital of all Russian Music, and a juried concert conducted with choir and orchestra.

I always planned to be an ear surgeon. That ran in the family – my father was one of the original ear surgeons – and I had not planned on practicing voice medicine. But as a professional singer, when I went to Michigan to do my residency, my music colleagues called me to find out what to do about their voice problems. I looked it up and there was almost nothing there. So, I started writing papers and books and doing research and met the few excellent people who were active in voice medicine, and helped develop a much needed new specialty. I wrote the first paper in the modern era teaching doctors how to take care of singers, and it was published in 1981. I also wrote the first chapter in an otolaryngology textbook, which was published in 1986, and then the first book on care of the voice which was published in 1991.

Now that was voice medicine. Arts medicine is a broader area that involves not just voice but hands, foot and ankle problems for dancers, and many other areas. That didn't really develop until the 1980s, and was spurred by colleagues named Alice Brandfonbrener, and Dick Lederman. The three of us met through mutual interests in arts medicine in general, and wrote the *Textbook of Performing Arts Medicine* in 1991, the first book on arts medicine which is now in its third edition.

Dr Gould had started The Voice Foundation Symposia in 1972, and I attended in 1977. We became fast friends instantaneously. He recognized my interest and appreciated the fact that I was in mainstream academic otolaryngology, which was important to the evolution of voice medicine. We started collaborating immediately which led to his inviting me to join the board of The Voice Foundation, eventually moving TVF to Philadelphia, and turning the Foundation over to me.

Linda M. Carroll, CCC-SLP, PhD, MPhil, MS

ASHA Fellow
Senior Voice Scientist: Otorhinolaryngology, The Children's Hospital of Philadelphia
Research Scientist: Otorhinolaryngology–Head and Neck Surgery, Montefiore Medical Center, Bronx, New York
Adjunct Professor: Music Business, New Jersey City University

My background is as a coloratura soprano. I had a double bachelors in voice – a bachelor in voice performance and a bachelor of science in music education – from University of Maine. In 1981, I moved to Philadelphia for a bad marriage, was busy singing with the Philadelphia Singers and some other places, and needed to get a job. We lived near Jefferson, as my then husband was working part-time there. We lived in the residence building, and someone there heard me singing and invited me to the Jefferson choir. They said, "We need sopranos" and I thought, "You need sopranos like a hole in the head!" but they said, "No, no, come!" Bob was the conductor.

So I started singing in the choir, and was working part time in Jefferson in the physiology/cardiology department, going through publications to find out who was the author and requesting reprints. At a rehearsal in January 1982, Bob asked me if I wanted a job. He was looking for a full time front desk administration/receptionist, handling a switchboard of seven lines. Shortly thereafter an assistant left suddenly and I was dealing with everything by myself. I took over the front desk, helped with the accounts, with the transcriptions, and helped with the audiologist. Down in the basement, there began to emerge a pulmonary lab, acoustics lab, ENG room and a special procedures room.

I started my Masters in speech pathology at Temple, and had an agreement with them that they would not ask me to stop singing, and that they understood I worked in a medical practice. One semester from graduation, the faculty gave me a no-confidence vote because they had significant concerns about how much time I was spending singing and seeing people for voice. They also thought that working in a medical practice was giving an abnormal slant to my view of speech pathology. This was in 1989, or 1990 and at that time, the speech pathology program was in the school of psychology. They asked me, "If someone is referred to you for voice, what is the first thing you want to know?" And I said, "I want to know what their larynx looks like." They said, "Wrong. You need to know their psychological profile." So I left the program. A year later I decided to finish the Masters elsewhere and go for that, and a PhD at Columbia. So, in 1991, I moved from Philadelphia to NYC, doing a double Masters and PhD at Columbia University, starting in January 1992 (under the mentorship of Ron Baken).

William Riley

Master Teacher: Voice, New Jersey City University

I had been working at Westminster Choir College full time and won a number of international voice competitions, then made the decision to become a freelancer instead of a college professor. During the time that I was flexible, Dr Gould said that he would like me to do voice evaluations in his voice practice, and I thought that would be something for a part-time person to do that would not interfere with academic issues, so I started doing that in 1989. My job there was not clearly defined and meant a lot of things. Basically, one of the things I had to do a lot of was work with the Recording and Research Center for the

Denver Center for the Performing Arts and The Voice Foundation. I was living in Princeton and commuting to work with Dr Gould until 1990, when I moved to New York.

Essentially my job in New York was similar to Linda Carroll's in Philadelphia. As a voice teacher, I was doing patient evaluations of the voice and communicating with Linda about various things that Gould wanted to have at the next Symposium. If the people he would send down the hall to me for evaluation had never had a voice lesson, I would give them an initial session, but my job was to find them someone in the community. If they didn't already have a teacher, I would refer them to one. So I got to know who all the good teachers and all the bad teachers were, and I would refer these patients to teachers who could help them.

Linda and I were constantly communicating and we had already begun dating. We were not only singing teachers with our own practices, but we were similar in other ways. Now we would also be called Medical Assistants, as we assisted with different procedural things in the practice. At that time, Linda was not yet a speech pathologist. When she decided to do that, Bob Sataloff was not so happy because it meant he had to lose her daily presence in his Philadelphia practice.

Vija Dale was Gould's secretary, and she liked me because I calmed down Dr Gould. Even patients commented that for that last four or five years of his life he was a much calmer, saner person. He could have a strong temper. Jim would calmly and discreetly demand that you jump.

Mary J. Hawkshaw, RN, BSN, CORLN

Research Associate Professor: Otolaryngology–Head and Neck Surgery, Drexel University College of Medicine
Executive Director: American Institute of Voice and Ear Research

I joined Dr Sataloff's practice completely by accident! I had done critical care nursing, open-heart surgery, and was head nurse of an open-heart ICU for ten years. I was pursuing an MSN MBA at Penn and Wharton when I realized that I didn't want a career path in business or nursing administration. I took a year off and did a lot of skiing, fashion design, and floral design – things I enjoyed. Then Dr Sataloff's first partner, who I'd known since he was in medical school, contacted me because they needed another nurse. What do you think? Will you come join us? And I said, "Oh my gosh a doctor's office, after fast-track critical care . . . I don't know, but I'll give you six months." And that was in 1986.

Three weeks after I started with them, Dr Sataloff's nurse left the practice and I became the nurse for both doctors and Dr Joseph Sataloff, Bob's father, who was still in practice! The practice was booming, and it got to the point where we needed another nurse to handle three doctors, so we looked at the needs of the practice. I already had done a lot of ghostwriting and editing, so that's when I became more dedicated to Bob and to his practice and helped him pioneer the field of laryngology.

Back then, we were just getting the *Journal of Voice* off the ground. When I started, we were just doing the transcriptions of the Symposia. But then we started the *Journal of Voice* and when you start a new journal you're desperately trying to get articles – I used to get so many Chinese submissions in questionable English and I had to re-write them. That's how my ghostwriting began.

I had never considered myself a good writer at all; I dreaded term papers and all that. But Dr Sataloff has a way of recognizing talent in people that they don't necessarily know they have. He is an extraordinary teacher, devoted to education.

So, I began writing for him and he would then edit what I wrote. I learned from him and also worked closely with parent publishers. Then I helped him with the first *Laryngology* textbook in 1991. It's no small feat doing these textbooks! And I've co-authored, eight or ten books, probably close to three hundred articles, and numerous book chapters.

Since becoming affiliated with Drexel College of Medicine, I have worked closely with our residents, medical students and fellows, assisting them in writing for publication, how to do their research, how to do literature reviews and coordinate all their studies. I also serve as the research coordinator for any study that's going on in our practice. In the meantime, through the years, I've worn many, many hats.

There was a time when I was the Symposium Coordinator; I've always been involved. I help with deciding on the program, what is going to be focused on, which papers are going to be selected, making sure there's the proper balance between medical, vocology, pedagogy, and voice science. And I'm a member of the Symposium planning committee, which meets on the last day of every Symposium – there are about six of us – and we decide the topic for next year and potential keynote speakers, G. Paul Moore lecturers, so forth.

9

Educating Each Other

> You need to reveal that you are communicating something very important and something very funny and interesting. That's the entrance ticket to communication, I think.
>
> J. Sundberg, PhD

R. C. Scherer, PhD: The primary aspect of the Symposia that has changed over the many years, is that the education and the knowledge base of all the attendees is so much broader and deeper now. At the beginning, there was a desire for each of the disciplines to make sure their own discipline was enhanced, and we had poor skills in communicating across disciplines.

That is absolutely reversed now at the Symposia. There are highly interactive discussions and questions by everybody, no matter the discipline, so that the emotions aren't relative to defending a discipline, but reflect passions to know more eclectically. People want to know what other disciplines are doing and what the latest ideas and findings are, because they know that they will do their jobs better with this information.

I think that is the primary reason why people go to the Symposia, as well as to see friends. You know, the voice community is not the largest community in the world, and it's really good to go to certain meetings and symposia where your colleagues and friends are, where you get recharged with energy and new ideas.

H. M. Tucker, MD: I think the organization is instrumental in the fact that young researchers who might otherwise not get a hearing anywhere can get a hearing by bringing a poster. So, because young people who do not yet have big credentials can get into the program at the Symposia much easier than they can get on the podium of some of the big national or international specialty societies, the Symposia have provided a fertile ground for young people to bring their new ideas. It is also where people of disparate backgrounds can get together, and someone from Hungary might come with an idea that someone from Chicago hears and says, "Wow, that fits in with what I have been doing" and they get together this way.

It's always, always stimulating. It's never boring, and coincident to all of that, is that the people who are there on a regular basis, for whatever reason, end up being very pleasant people to interact with, and I have developed a couple of international friendships that continue outside of the Symposia for various reasons.

———

B. Raphael, PhD: The team approach to treating a voice is much more common today than it was when I first got involved, and would hear, "Why are you going to a voice symposium?" and think, "What am I here for? I'm an actor! I'm a teacher. I spend my time in the theater and I coach people in plays and in performance. What are you going to that scientific thing for?" And to the scientists I would be sort of a pseudo-scientist, because I wasn't a real scientist – I was a theater person.

One reason Ron Scherer and I got along so well and did really good work together, in my opinion, is that he respected my side of the town and I respected his. And the whole is greater than the sum of the parts. So, the biggest change I have seen is the team approach. When somebody comes in with a voice problem, it's not just a doctor looking down their throat and writing a prescription or advising surgery. We talk about nutrition, we talk about lifestyle, we talk about how to warm-up when you're well, how to warm-up when you're sick, if you have just so much energy.

———

J. Sundberg, PhD: So, The Voice Foundation meetings are the leading, the main forum for new voice research, I think. Voice research in its own right.

Tom Shipp came to Sweden, he was friends with a colleague in my lab, and he probably had seen some article of mine. 1977 . . . that could have been the *Scientific American* perhaps. So, then I was invited to go there and to speak about my research on the singer's formant, I think.

Tom Shipp was very warm and a good person, he took care of me and made me feel comfortable in this very, very new and unfamiliar setting. And then it was great to meet all these people who you have been quoting in your work. See them and talk with them.

I remember talking with Tom Hixon and he mentioned to me the tracheal pull; the force that the trachea is exerting on the larynx trying to pull it down and trying to abduct the vocal folds, and we talked about that in a break. Then I was contacted by phoniatrician-singer Rolf Leanderson, and he wanted to do research together with me. And I contacted Curt von Euler, who was a physiologist and a wonderful guy, and top quality researcher. So we started to team up and measured the breathing apparatus. The tracheal pull was also the topic of two doctoral dissertations, one by singing teacher Monica Thomasson, and the other by speech and language therapist Jenny Iwarsson.

That talk with Tom Hixon was the most important thing in the development of my research – and that was due to a talk at the Symposium. And, I think, this is typical of what happens in Symposia. You get contacts and you get stimulating talks; you get ideas and you can test your own ideas with those of other people who have tried that before, or maybe they want to go there. So Symposia are exceedingly important for maintaining and defending quality research.

———

P. Woo, MD: In those early years, it was very helpful. By going to the Symposia, you sort of had a lay of the land, by going to that one Symposium every year, you could get a pretty good idea of where the world of voice is. What they know, and eventually, as you yourself became more sophisticated, an idea of what they don't know. It was always helpful, because you could see that they don't know that much about this or that, and maybe we should look at it from this direction or that. So it was helpful in stimulating projects.

During the early years, the scientific director, David Brewer, one of the early founders of TVF, was at Syracuse with us. We would talk about projects and new ideas after the Symposia, which was really helpful. We had one of the early voice teams, which are stressed at TVF.

TVF is a wonderful banner for people in voice and continues to be so today. You see people come from all over the world to gather, SLPs, singing teachers, medical people, it is not easy. Most meetings are more specialized. TVF continues to be like this umbrella that gets people to come together and talk about multiple aspects, which was one of the initial goals of Jim Gould when he started TVF, which is terrific.

M. Benninger, MD: There's always some new science, some new voice therapy options, there's some good free papers, and some really nice posters. I think that the most enjoyable part of the Symposium is going to the Friday afternoon tutorials, where I actually can see how the singers and the vocal teachers approach their art. This is much more instructive to me than the medical science portion, which I can get in other forums. I also think the poster session is just great because it is a lot of young people from all over the world for whom this is their first time presenting.

The Voice Foundation is a nice blend of the premier people in the world dedicated to voice health, with different knowledge backgrounds, and coming from different cultures through the various subspecialties that participate in the program. The young people new to the Symposium tend to look up to those of us that have been around for a while and it creates interesting discussions and interactions. Another thing that I really, really enjoy about the program is getting an opportunity to sit and kind of challenge their ideas, try to stimulate them to do more research, and to learn how these young, vibrant minds are going to expand our specialty.

It is also where I've met a good number of my non-physician colleagues from around the world, some of whom I've subsequently published with, some of whom I've done research with, and some of whom I've visited and done social things with. For several people, I have been one of their PhD thesis advisors.

R.J. Baken, PhD: On the one hand, our Symposia keep our various professionals up to date on developments and controversies in their specialties, and in our collective enterprise. On the other hand, the Symposia encourage more people (and, one hopes, especially our colleagues in the vocal arts) to get involved in systematic research. We know that there are still arts people out there who are fiercely opposed to research in voice. One of the things that the Symposia do is give a home to those people in the musical community who are in favor it. There are even a number of prominent singing teachers I can think of who have become passionate about serious research in singing, very much in the spirit and footsteps of William Vennard. I believe that The Voice Foundation can be very proud of that.

J. LoVetri: I was referred to the Symposium by a speech pathologist and I stumbled, literally stumbled, into some lectures, and I remember at the time being really excited about what I was seeing. It was the first time I had attended a conference on the voice, and I was thrilled to see people talking about the larynx and vocal folds. I was also very ignorant, and knew that I had a lot to learn in order to be able to benefit from the research being presented there.

It was a stimulus for me to read books on vocal production. I would have a small glimmer of hope to understand things better in subsequent years. I began to be able to ask questions of presenters during the breaks, and people were very kind and answered them. I met more participants and began to create a personal network within The Voice Foundation community and this was very helpful to me as well.

Some of the people involved in the early Voice Foundation Symposia who brought me into the fold, were Dr Lucille Rubin, who really extended herself to me and was extraordinarily kind; Dr Alan Keaton who was an ENT from Seattle; Dr Ingo Titze, and Dr Ron Scherer. Also I was assisted at the sessions by some of the speech pathologists, young women like me, who guided me through anything that had to do with research related to speech or vocal function, and explained a little bit more about the charts and graphs I was seeing.

Gradually, I got to know, at least minimally, a lot of the core people who were involved in the Symposium at that time and, as I got more exposure to their work, I understood all the information more completely. Many of these professionals would answer whatever questions I had, which was very kind of them, because I probably asked very stupid basic questions!

―――――――――

M. Behlau, PhD: What I took home into my practice was the model – the teamwork model. We were already working on teamwork here with my director, Professor Pontes, but I took home another level of teamwork, which was tolerance of others' perspectives. So, it really opened my mind, my eyes. My panorama was broadened by The Voice Foundation and what I took back home was the excellence level that The Voice Foundation cherishes. It wants to do everything on an excellent level. The panel, the coffee break, the name badge, the stripes with colors, the secretary, the master class, the gala. So, they search for nothing less than excellence. Nothing but the best. And I took this back home. You should do your best. You should be there. So, I think that The Voice Foundation makes you want to come back. If you go there once, you get hooked.

I owe my post-doctoral appointment to The Voice Foundation too. One year, a famous surgeon called Herbert Dedo from California, was making a presentation at a Symposium and he had a very severe round table, a very harsh fight with Professor Aronson from the Mayo Clinic about a surgery on spasmodic dysphonia. After that, I talked to him on my experience in Brazil, and Professor Dedo invited me to join him to do a post-doctoral fellowship at University of California, San Francisco. So, due to The Voice Foundation, I got a position in California and went to a one-year post-doctoral fellowship with my baby son, Thomas. We were there during the 1989 earthquake, so I had this very exciting experience of surviving an earthquake in the Bay area!

I also manage to have my students working and studying with other professors in the US due to The Voice Foundation. So, The Voice Foundation not only helped me with my education, but also helps my students, and offers opportunities to my students to go and exchange information with the other American colleagues. It is a powerful networking strategy!

―――――――――

H. M. Tucker, MD: Well, you understand that it is fairly recent, to be honest, that we are able to communicate across the ocean with colleagues. There are several reasons for it: Getting out from under the horrible effects of World War II took at least twenty years, and it was not until the 1980s that there was any communication at all behind the Iron Curtain. Then, obviously, changes in long-distance telephone communication, the growth of the internet and the ability to Skype all, indirectly, have a lot to do with where we are with this organization.

The Voice Foundation was truly one of the first international organizations in which people from outside the United States would take part, which was beneficial in two ways. It was not only beneficial to them, but it allowed us to become au courant with some of the innovations taking place in Europe, India, Japan, and China. There is a lot going on around the world in every type of medical specialty, and particularly in ours. TVF has been instrumental in developing interaction and communication and for want of a better term, friendships, among the educators around the world who have an interest in voice. And this has been a huge benefit.

―――――――――

B. Raphael, PhD: I also really felt badly for the fact that there were Japanese people there, and there were Swedish presenters. So, the Japanese attendees and presenters are trying to understand this very technical material, presented in English with a Swedish accent. So, for years, to many people's annoyance, I was constantly pleading for translators or interpreters at the end of each day's presentations at The Voice Foundation to put it in layman's terms for those of us who just got lost.

———

M. Behlau, PhD: When I was first attending the Symposia, I didn't dare to present, but I told Professor Sataloff, "We have this new surgery on sulcus vocalis, proposed by Prof. Paulo Pontes." And he said, "Why don't you come and present" and I said, "Me?! No, I don't think so." And he said, "No, no, no. You present, I'll help you." So I wrote the paper. My English was terrible. So he said, "An anonymous reviewer worked on your paper." And I said, "Oh, Professor, tell me who was the anonymous reviewer because I have to send a gift." He said, "I was the anonymous reviewer." He, himself, rewrote it entirely to transfer it into plain English. That was my first *Journal of Voice* paper.

For my first presentation, I was on the podium because Professor Sataloff took me there. He was in front of me and just waving, go, go, go, go. I was terrified. I was trembling. I was suffering a lot. And he said "Go." It was a surgery paper, presented by a Brazilian SLP with limited English, so it was . . . it was hard. But everybody liked it. The surgery was accepted in the US, and they started performing it. And that gave me the confidence I needed to move forward.

———

It takes courage to present in front of the formidable, diverse audience at the Symposia. Even more courage when the presentation is in a foreign language that you use only occasionally and that doesn't fit your tongue well. When that language is American English, which delights in breaking its rules of pronunciation, and whose grammatical rules are a moving target, the task can be daunting. Then, even when you have practiced your speech, there are the questions to be answered and, suddenly, one can be in a quagmire of linguistic spontaneity.

Free Presentation Coaching is offered at the Symposia through the Presentation Outreach program. Top level coaches donate their time to work with presenters on 'Turning great data into a solid presentation.' These half-hour sessions are available to all presenters, although many foreign presenters do not know to ask for coaching, or feel they couldn't add anything else to their plate in the moment. And many native speakers do not realize how much they could benefit. Those who have utilized the coaches have found them very helpful and have had outstanding results.

———

R. J. Baken, PhD: *Do you think the Symposia have raised a generation of people who can present?* To speak to each other, yes. That shows very clearly, for instance, in some of the discussions with poster-presentation authors. But have we raised a generation of good speakers? No. They may not be any worse than the speakers of years ago, but all too many are no better – in spite of the fact that technology now provides so many aids to effective communication. We offer coaching to those who want it, but I wish there were some way we could insist on it for some of our participants. It would be nice to be able to say, "You have great ideas, but it is painful watching you. You should do something about that."

———

How often is it, that in lecturing, performing, or demonstrating we focus on whether or not we are getting it right or doing well, rather than on our own fascination with the information we are presenting? Dr Sundberg's following observations were brought to life for the author on an airplane, when within several sentences of the flight attendant's safety instructions, everyone went quiet and gave her their full attention. Not because she was amusing, but because she was riveting. It would have been supremely rude to ignore her. She made it clear to bored, tired travelers that this mundane, oft-repeated information was fascinating and very important.

———

J. Sundberg, PhD: It is most interesting in Symposia to sit and listen to how people try to communicate what they are saying. Some people are excellent presenters and you feel that this is very important and very interesting, so you get absorbed. Other people get absorbed by their nerves, and they are so nervous that it turns out to be a communication between the manuscript and the presenter, who considers the audience as sort of irrelevant.

It is the same act of communication which you have in music, in lecturing and in acting. When you communicate, you need to make it clear to the listener that this is very, very fascinating and interesting, and that I'm burning to communicate this with you. If this is missing, no communication takes place. It's just a little rest time for the audience.

This is exactly what I have been working with around music performance and the principles that are being applied in musical performance. You need to reveal that you are communicating something very important and something very funny and interesting. That's the entrance ticket to communication, I think.

10

Philadelphia

> The Symposia foster cross-disciplinary understanding, collaboration, deeper thinking about one's own questions, and long-term friendships that stimulate future harmony within the professions.
>
> R.C. Scherer, PhD

R. C. Scherer, PhD: Relative to The Voice Foundation, our mission – to bring the disciplines together for the advancement of voice, especially for those who apply and use the voice – has never been altered, and has only been augmented.

G. Korovin, MD: Dr Gould realized he was getting older and not able to fully run it, and didn't really have the resources to fully do what he wanted to do with it. I think he realized he couldn't financially keep it going. He was making plans for who was going to keep this going, Bob was very involved with it, and Bob felt he could run it more easily through his office.

M. Hawkshaw, CORLN: Dr Gould passed the reins on to Dr Sataloff in 1989, and the Symposium moved to Philadelphia.

The mission of TVF did not change; it just kept growing and growing. But running it changed in a big way, most of all because it had no known presence in Philadelphia and Dr Gould had a lot of very wealthy patrons in New York. He was a good fundraiser, and the galas were galas. I mean, they were huge and elaborate, with prominent attendees in the worlds of acting, singing, opera, finance, politics, broadcasting and 'high society'. It was a very well-endowed foundation in New York City, so it was like starting anew here in Philadelphia, where we weren't a known commodity and we didn't have all the patrons. Some of them followed. Leon Fassler remained extremely active, which kept things running.

W. Riley: At that point, Sataloff had an expanding cadre of speech and voice staff and administrative staff that all worked together as a team, as a single unit, always trying to make things work. Sataloff's team was all in one office, whereas Gould's team was spread out all over the country. The two practices were very different in that aspect. Gould's hospital was far away, and he no longer served as the head of laryngology at Lenox Hill, although he still had a laboratory there (the Voice Dynamics Laboratory). But he was involved with NIH to a great extent, the NCVS to a great extent, and president of TVF. Gould had groomed Sataloff to be his successor and there came a moment, during the two or three years of transition, when Jim Gould would have Sataloff up to his practice quite often, for a new business venture: EPIC (Executive Performance In Voice Training) and eventually the transfer of The Voice Foundation to Sataloff took place. At that point Linda Carroll was the point man for a lot of things in Sataloff's office (voice training, voice lab measures, TVF, *Journal Of Voice*, and music events). When she left to pursue her PhD in 1991, she was replaced with five people.

L. Carroll, CCC-SLP: The support staff in Philadelphia were used to working with each other all the time, so there was a greater ability to keep track of everything, catch things as they were falling, and keep them from other people's eyes. In New York, it was some people from Jim's office, some people from here, some people from there, who would only work together at Symposium time. In Philadelphia, the team was already in sync.

The first Symposium in Philadelphia was at Hotel Atop the Bellevue. That's where the outbreak of Legionnaire's disease had been. They had revamped the whole hotel, making a major renovation. The Symposium was occurring two weeks after they had re-opened the hotel. It was very risky. They had had one event in their major ballroom, but nothing as large and involved as the Symposium, especially with as tight a schedule as TVF needs. Fifteen minutes behind can create serious problems.

For this first Symposium at Hotel Atop the Bellevue, the lighting company was from Manayunk, a Philadelphia suburb. It was complicated because in that venue we had to use rear projection slides, so each slide needed to be turned and reversed. We had AV come in and set the rear projection and reset the light boards, and they finished setting everything at 1:00 am. Then we all came back at 5:30 in the morning, and AV came in and all the slide projectors were gone. All the cables were missing. The lights had been re-programmed back to their original setting. Not a small feat in three or four hours.

Meanwhile we have the first paper at 8 am. Fortunately, the AV contractor's warehouse in Manayunk was nearby. They dispatched a truck filled up with slide projectors and cables and started restructuring it all. Meanwhile faculty was showing up and needing to reset all their slides because of the rear-projection.

The hotel had no idea where all the equipment had gone. The police got involved, and on the last day they found all the equipment upstairs, on an upper floor, in the administrative offices in a locked cabinet.

Bob had chosen this beautiful site and really wanted to convince Jim that it was going to be OK. At the hotel, it was one thing after another: first the AV was disastrous, then catering missed the 20 minute coffee break by 15 minutes and they were having trouble being quiet enough. After that experience, the Symposium moved to the Warwick Hotel.

Alice McHugh used to run the Symposia for Jim, so when I first came on, I was Alice's assistant. Alice didn't work in his office, but she coordinated the Symposia from the very beginning. Then I became Symposium Coordinator, which involves collecting the abstracts. Bob decides which division they go to, they are mailed off to the heads of that division, at which point they are ranked in order and returned to the office by the beginning of December (the abstract deadline was, and still is, October 31).

Bob and I would lay them all out, and I would type the entire program between Christmas and New Year. Personal computers had just come out. Then it would go off to print, be proofed, and be ready for mailing by February 14th. That was Jim Gould's rule. No matter what, out by February 14th, with mailing labels from AAO, ASHA and NATS, and at that time mass mailings needed to be pre-stamped and sorted by region before going to the Post Office.

Starting around March 5th, Jim would call every

couple of days. "Hi, Linda, how are the registrations coming?" I needed to tell him how many MDs had registered, how many speech pathologists, how many voice teachers, what the cash flow was doing, what was outstanding. Everything went through Jim.

———

In November of 1985, Alice McHugh retired as Executive Director of The Voice Foundation, a position she had held for eight years. The March 1986 TVF Newsletter notes: "Under Alice's tutelage the Foundation grew from a dream, to be the nationally recognized source of information on vocal health and use. Her work developed the annual Symposium to the position of respect it now commands. […] Above all, it was Alice's hard work and persistent cheeriness which made the annual Gala such a success." The position of Executive Director was filled by Gary Gatza, a lawyer with extensive non-profit experience, and Linda Carroll took over as the first of a series of Symposium Coordinators.

———

G. Korovin, MD: When I started in 1989, I had just missed a meeting (because of my residency) and Gould said, "Oh, you'll be there next year." I remember him on the phone talking about who would be attending, and going back and forth to Philadelphia on the train – he would attend and then return to look at some patients. By the weekend, he would stay over.

Indeed, he would call Philadelphia several times a day, keeping track of everything and how many people were attending.

———

Dr Gould recognized in Dr Sataloff the person who would continue the vision of interdisciplinary cooperation and give The Voice Foundation Symposia academic traction through his dedication to education and the dissemination of information, his rigorous scholarship and high standards.

———

C.R. Stasney, MD: I think the world of Bob Sataloff, and immediately say that he is the gold standard to which we all aspire. The things he's done to publicize scientific papers about voice care are just irreplaceable.

———

L. Rubin, PhD: As Jim let go of his surgery work, and died unexpectedly, the organization was literally saved by Dr Robert T. Sataloff. Bob transformed Jim Gould's fan club into a professional organization. Today, TVF has exceeded Jim's dreams thanks to the extraordinary vision and leadership of Dr Sataloff. He has taken TVF to the global stage while his miraculous Executive Director, Maria Russo, has enlisted a new, young membership that will keep TVF growing. Today there is a James Gould Award, offered in his memory and as an incentive to walk in Jim's footsteps.

———

L. Carroll, CCC-SLP: The attendance dropped after Jim's death. I think it was a combination of Jim not being there – and he had really been the drawing force for so many people – plus a shift in research away from talking about how to do surgery, into much more detailed work on the physiology of phonation, and research in the diseases that would have an impact on voice function. In those days, there were large disagreements around these subjects. For example, when the idea that reflux laryngitis existed and affected the voice was put forth by Jamie Koufman, it was summarily dismissed. A couple of years later, when she introduced the idea that vocal fold paresis existed, it was not considered a major issue or a common concern, and it too was dismissed. Today these concepts are both considered major diagnostic challenges in the arena of elite voice care.

There was the "Why can't you just bring it back to New York?" group, who liked to come to New York to see shows. Speech pathology was starting a little bit of voice, there were not many speech pathology and voice combos, voice teachers were threatened by the science, and there are not as many teachers in Philadelphia as New York. In Manhattan, the teachers would stop in and bring their students with them. There would be a hundred and twenty-five walk-ins a day. You don't get that in Philadelphia.

M. Behlau, PhD: Sometimes it's hard at first because, well, it's Philadelphia: no direct flight, they are too conservative, too traditional, too 'Philadelphia', too American-oriented. And then you arrive there, and people are warm and open, and they help and they make you feel comfortable. And everybody from the staff – the staff is a real jewelry box – but, besides the staff, even the audio-visual people that are always the same, they come back every year, they call me by my name. They always say, "Hi, Mara. We know you're going to have irregular files on audio, we will fix that." So we know it all, so they make you feel like home.

Executive Director Maria Russo is . . . I have no words to tell about her because she is so focus-oriented, she is so stable and her level of attention is so high towards everybody. She makes all of us feel at home.

Anthony 'Tony' Lambiase recorded the first Symposia on reel-to-reel tape, and remained as the AV Administrator through the first couple of years in Philadelphia, helping smooth the Symposia's transition. Sharon Radionoff held the reins in 1991, then Margaret 'Peggy' Baroody took over as the Audio-Visual Coordinator and has been one of the Symposia mainstays for over twenty years. Returning presenters already know they are in excellent hands, and that all will be well. The first-timers, wired and scared before their first presentation, encounter Peggy's remarkable equanimity and calm, and a level of fear sloughs off of them. One has to look closely to notice that behind that ease, all manner of sticks, thumb-drives, and computer files fly past, feeding simultaneous, uninterrupted chains of presentations changing every fifteen minutes in two rooms.

Then there are the sudden changes in the dance card, when a presenter is confused by jet lag, suddenly delayed by weather, in hospital, giving birth, or just mysteriously not there when they should be. It is a very impressive magic act, without which the Symposium would quickly grind to a clumsy halt. (It should be noted that the presenter giving birth did manage to forward her PowerPoint to Peggy, and the talk was presented.)

Margaret Baroody: The quality of our AV company, Projections, and their extraordinary, professional staff are the key to the success we might feel that we achieve. Each member of the AV team is willing to go above and beyond to make every presentation a success. I may be the facilitator but the AV guys are what make it all happen.

I have been the official AV coordinator since 1992. That was in the days of slides, which were a difficult process to coordinate. Between the loading and unloading of slides, the lack of enough slide trays, the problems with the slides themselves . . . ***yipes***!

I have always been a true believer in the very critical role The Voice Foundation has played in advancing the care of the voice. So many voice professionals owe their career to the ever-expanding knowledge and treatment modalities regarding voice, that are a direct result of the collaborative, educational and inspirational impact of the Symposium. Getting to know the wonderful returning attendees over the years, as well as meeting new people, is a constant source of inspiration.

R.J. Baken, PhD: I don't know that we saw a sharp division in the move to Philadelphia. I think Bob Sataloff shares Jim Gould's point of view, and with that shared perspective there has been continuity. Any good tradition evolves over time. We have more constituencies now, and we try as best we can to address all of their – sometimes very different – needs. One important change has been that we now split part of the meeting by professional group. One of Jim Gould's adamant points was that singers have to be there to hear the medical people, and medical people need to sit there and listen to the singers because we need to talk to each other. Now it has become more and more necessary to let people escape and be with their own professional cohort. To some extent, that's because things have gotten so technical – on both sides – that 'outsiders' struggle. Also, people want to get information that is of immediate relevance to them; and there is so much information now, that it's utterly impractical to try to fit it into one meeting.

I do remember that, in the days when I participated in the program committee for the Symposia, there was long, heavy, and soul-searching debate about the wisdom of a divided meeting. Ultimately it became clear that it had to happen.

Round-table discussions can be problematic: There are always going to be people, especially in the audience, who are fanatics and will either try to dominate a discussion, or move it into off-topic areas. One needs a strong moderator who will tell such individuals, when necessary, to sit down. We are, all of us, acculturated not to do that. But the role of the moderator is to maintain focus – a tricky undertaking. There must be the understanding, I think, that a strong moderator is going to provoke occasional complaints to management.

C.R. Stasney, MD: I started going in the late 1980s, in New York, then was there pretty much every year that Bob has had it. I may not be a great speaker, but I'm a great moderator, Bob used to call me all the time, kind of like the minister calls you to acolyte in church because you haven't shown up in awhile? He would call me and say, "Could you moderate this panel?" And these personalities on the panel would be unbelievable. But when I'm moderating something, if somebody has seven minutes to give a presentation, then that's what they got. By George, I cut it off. That's it. Next . . . ? I was trying to make sure that everybody, even the quiet people, got their say on a panel.

C. Sapienza, PhD: When I first started attending the Symposia it was intimidating! All the biggies, whatever name you could think of, were all there attending and they didn't make it easy on podium presenters. They called you out a lot more than people do today. They could've picked on me a lot more, but they liked me; there were some people that were really kind, and they liked the work I was doing. Overall, there was a buzz, lots of activity, with Dr Bob Sataloff demonstrating lots of sophistication in the quality of the program and the organization of the program. It was intimidating, but in an exciting way.

Once, after presenting, I wanted to get Dr Christy Ludlow's attention to see how she liked my presentation. I was young and she probably didn't listen to me, to the detail that I thought she might, and she didn't give me quite that crisp feedback I was looking for, but I remember getting those couple of minutes with her just to get a little bit of a validation. Now we are great friends and colleagues. She treated me like she should have, making me work to earn my stripes. I remember my first presentation at a Symposium in 1990, because I had typed the whole thing out and I read it. Later on that same day, Dr Christy Ludlow gave hers without reading it, and it was just par excellence. I remember asking her, "How do you do that without reading?" She said, "You'll get there. You just have to know your work really well." And I think after that presentation, I never read mine again. I saw how she did it and thought, boy, reading it is too structured; it's not flexible, it's not creative. So, I worked really hard to never read my presentation after that.

I can't think of one thing from the Symposia I didn't take back home with me. I learned how to present. I learned how to interact with peers and colleagues. I learned how to ask appropriate questions. I learned how to be a part of a panel discussion. I learned about grant funding. I was asked to be part of the *Journal of Voice* Editorial Board. I learned how to serve on a board. I learned how to be a part of peer review. I participated in organizing parts of the conference. I brought my own students there to present and to integrate their work into The Voice Foundation. I learned how to capitalize on the social moments that you have, and how to socialize and bring work in at the right times, and how to leave it out at other times.

K. Ardo: During those early Symposia, there were breakout rooms where they would go over case studies. Most of the people in the room were otolaryngologists, and Dr Sataloff would first play the voice of the person that was in the case study, without showing anything else. The next question would be, "Who would like to say what they hear?" and, young and naïve, my hand just went up and I'd say, "Well I think this person has something wrong on the left side of his vocal cords and I hear this and I hear that." Dr Sataloff would always be stupefied that, before they showed the clinical study, the actual picture of what was going on in that person, my hand was always going up and saying what I heard, because I have this amazing perception of being able to pick up what is happening in another person's body.

Maybe, because of all the years of muscle memory in my own body, I'm able to pick these things up much more quickly and perceive them just by hearing the voice. I don't know how I have this gift. That's beyond me, but I just know that everybody was pretty much stunned, that here was this young person always jumping up, eager to say what they heard without seeing examples of what's going on, and being right all the time.

This was very early on in the first or second year after the Symposia moved to Philadelphia, and I think that helped to formulate my friendship with Dr Sataloff – that kind of drew us together: his interest in finding out what makes Katherine tick, how is she able to do that? It also emboldened me, and gave me more confidence when people approached me and started talking to me, welcomed me into the conferences, and took seriously my interest and my amazing perception abilities of hearing what was going on.

This has also proved invaluable to me when I am working with certain ear, nose, and throat specialists. We have a different medical system here. You need to be referred by your family physician and then, sometimes, it takes up to three months to get an appointment. That doesn't work with professional people that are on the road and trying to keep their careers going. If I phone the ENTs about somebody, they know that there is something happening; that if I'm calling, there is something wrong with that person and they'd better find the time.

R. H. Colton, PhD: The Voice Foundation has performed a yeoman's task over the years of bringing disparate groups together. There are other meetings now, but Jim and others started it. Jim Gould had a very far-sighted view of what he wanted to do and what the Symposia should be. If you talked to him now, I think he would be very pleased with how it is all going. His successor, Bob Sataloff, has continued the effort to bring all these groups together and expanded the scope of the mission. It was the meeting I always wanted to go to because there was so much about voice. You get a little voice other places, but The Voice Foundation is all about the voice, and you get the latest information, and information that hasn't even been published yet. You get a sense for what people are thinking about the voice from numerous perspectives.

H. Blackwell: I was honored and gave a masterclass about four or five years ago, and the experience was remarkable. The Symposium was remarkable. I didn't have enough time to attend every session – I was hoping to double or treble myself, to attend every session. I was there for two days. The wealth of information being presented was astounding, not only scientifically but practically. I thought that was very helpful to the aspect of teaching. I was able to take back several things into the studio from the sessions I attended, especially a session about jaw tension that really helped. Each subsequent year, I've been thinking that this is the year I'm going back, but I've been performing during that period.

J. LoVetri: In 2006, Dr Sataloff scheduled the very first contemporary commercial music pedagogy panel at the Symposium. It felt to me then, that all the commercial styles were now being accepted for research – we wanted to look at them, and we wanted to encourage young people to look at them. That panel consisted of Dr Sundberg, Dr Sataloff, Robert Edwin, Dr Doug Hicks of The Cleveland Clinic, and Dominique Eade, a former student of mine, who runs the jazz vocal department at New England Conservatory. The panel consisted of two singing teachers (one music theater and CCM, the other one jazz), as well as a medical doctor, a clinical doctor and a research doctor. I was the moderator. It was the last thing on the Symposium program, scheduled to run for half an hour, but Dr Sataloff allowed it to go another twenty or twenty-five minutes longer. It was very successful.

Subsequently, Dr Sataloff allowed me to write an Editorial about contemporary commercial music in the *Journal of Voice*. That seemed to me to be an imprimatur of "Yes, we are now embracing CCM styles on an equal platform with classical styles, and research can commence in a serious manner." In 2015, many different styles are respected at the Symposium, and I think that's an outgrowth of the panel in 2006, and of Dr Sataloff's support of this music and the artists who sing it.

Looking to the Future

It is said that those who make a career in opera, especially a long career, are people who will not – cannot – be stopped. What does a well-respected and glorious-voiced Brünnhilde/Isolde/Elektra do when she is looking towards the next phase of her life? What could be challenging after Wagner and Strauss?

Maria Russo: Thanks to my friend and colleague from the Academy of Vocal Arts, Margaret (Peggy) Baroody, who knew that I was transitioning back to the US from a singing career abroad, and that I was looking for a new direction which would utilize my years of singing, opera theater and travel, I landed at The Voice Foundation in August 2010 as Executive Coordinator, with duties as the Managing Editor of *Journal of Voice* and assistant to the Executive Director. I enjoyed learning the process of publishing peer-reviewed articles for *Journal of Voice* from Dr Sataloff and, after three months, was settled into the job. I got to understand little by little, what determined a well-designed study and, even more, what made a thorough, considered peer-review.

The Voice Foundation had suffered the loss of grant money during the financial difficulties beginning in 2007 and by 2010, it had trickled down to small sponsorships. The circumstances became dire just as I entered the picture, and the extremely responsible Executive Director, at that time, felt that the only option was for her to resign and take the weight of two salaries off the organization. That's how I inherited the job of Director and was thrown into a 'do-or-die' situation.

The Voice Foundation, with its membership numbers and the size of the Symposium, should optimally be run by three full-time employees, but can, and does, function with two. Thoughts of me, just one untrained, full-time employee putting on the Symposium can still make me breathless, but as a working singer with a large performance repertoire, 'jumping in' to productions and performances at the last minute is the norm, especially in the

German-speaking countries. I have always loved that challenge.

Dr Sataloff is extremely practiced in Symposium-event planning and led me gently, step-by-step in everything, from A to Z. With panic calls to the former Director, the help of Symposium experts, Mary Hawkshaw, Margaret Baroody, the former Executive Coordinator, Julia Nawrocki, and helpers, Michelle Horman and David Pershica, and so many others, I learned about abstract submission, programming, food and beverage planning, hotel contracts, exhibitors, marketing and publicity, education credits, registration, etc., and everything you need to put on a Gala – in six easy months! The Symposium went off with only one major mistake among the usual problems that arise. Imagine my mortification, as the entire Editorial Board of *Journal of Voice* sat in the luncheon meeting waiting for the Publisher from Elsevier to give her yearly report and she wasn't even in the hotel. Hasty calls determined that, yes, I had given the Publisher of *Journal of Voice* the wrong date for the meeting.

It's a gift to be able to say that I love my job. The challenges keep me going; I am constantly delighted by what I learn from Dr Sataloff. Particularly in the first year, we would laugh as he would readjust my sentences back to good English from German sentence structure.

At the Symposia, it thrills me to watch the mystical aspects of singing and speech confront the definitions of science and medicine, and start to meet at the edges. I don't know anyone who can better articulate and realize this synthesis than Dr Sataloff. I believe in this organization and think that my biggest contribution is as a facilitator. Nancy Pearl Solomon and Ron Scherer have been such a big help to me in finding the way to make it happen.

Margaret Baroody: I suggested her for the position originally because of her intelligence and, although she did not have an administrative background, her computer skills combined with the many transferrable skills she possessed as a successful professional singer were enough, I believed, to give her a chance to succeed. And succeed she has! I have watched her bravely tackle an entire new career, and not only learn the job quickly, but have a tremendous influence on how The Voice Foundation now operates.

Using her social media skills, she has raised the public profile of the organization, attracting new members and supporters, and she has done it with very little budget. I cannot say enough about what Maria has brought to this organization. We should count ourselves lucky to have her.

M. Hawkshaw, CORLN: It is important to point out the continued interest in the success of the program. The folks that were there at the beginning are still there. Are still there. From otolaryngologists, to the voice scientists, the pedagogy folks to the singers. Year, after year, after year, they're back. They don't lose interest and they still understand the importance of these meetings.

And that's extremely exciting to me – that that has not waned over the years. And we're still cultivating new, young, scientists, and laryngologists. Things are tough now because of finances, of course; a lot of hospitals and academic institutions are limiting the number of conferences that physicians, employees, voice teachers, and scientists are able attend annually. That's impacted attendance, but the core people are still there, and that speaks to their dedication and commitment, so that's exciting.

L. Rubin, PhD: I'm pleased with the growing emphasis on the speaking voice, as it is now more frequently recognized and researched. Our Presentation Outreach committee has presented diverse voice methodologies into our Symposia workshops, that offer opportunities for scientific studies of the speaking voice. Voice needs will grow for the public speaker, actor, animated voice, impersonator, book narrator, voiceover artist, TV anchor, newscaster, legal and corporate presenter, teacher, physical exercise coach – and for all performing artists.

M. Behlau, PhD: I think that the possibility of sitting in an audience at The Voice Foundation with the luminaries in the field, who don't put themselves on a separate level, has been one of the main points. Everybody sits there, everybody makes presentations, everybody gets criticized. We laugh a lot. The foreigners are really funny, interesting and attractive – like Jean Abitbol, Josef Schlömicher-Thier, and Markus Hess, and all those people that have the strange accents – and we do dare, and we share our cultural things. But the way that people behave at The Voice Foundation is a friendship attitude, is a warm, colleague attitude. And the luminaries, the professors, they really, really like to help the students and the newcomers. I think this is unique. This is wonderful.

I think that the only thing that can make us stand out is to reinforce the uniqueness of the teamwork that is offered there. I think this is something. We need to attract more physicians, so I believe that they need to have special attention or a special strategy, such as surgical sessions, integration sessions, to have the physicians back, because they add a lot.

But, actually, I go to many international meetings and there is nothing that compares to The Voice Foundation. It is unique. I do see the struggle that has been happening these last years, I think we are doing better – newcomers, new people, larger attendance, but we need to work on online products to have profit.

M. Hawkshaw, CORLN: One point I want to make is the paucity of nurses that are involved in and attend these meetings. Almost zero. Dr Gould had a nurse – Kathy Yetman was her name. She was what I am to Bob, and she passed away, I think, a year or two before Dr Gould did. Kathy was very involved with TVF Symposia and I worked closely with her then.

Laryngologists and otolaryngologists probably have nurses, some have physician assistants, maybe nurse practitioners, medical assistants, and voice technologists, but they do not attend the meetings.

J. LoVetri: It would be nice to have one of the master classes at the symposium be a music theater master class and not an opera master class. It's time to diversify: bring in a Broadway celebrity and have them work with music theater singers, or have Vy Higginson do a gospel master class.

Perhaps, some kind of interfacing, interacting, think-tank kind of session where a doctor could ask somebody like Denyce Graves, "what did you mean?" I don't know how that could be managed in terms of times and space, but it would be an interesting dialog.

In the future, I would like The Voice Foundation to vet any sounds presented by researchers doing perceptual or pedagogical studies. Experienced experts who have their feet in the professional music marketplace need to hear and agree upon the sounds presented, and accept them as being representative of the music marketplace's professional expectations. This would prevent research not based on 'real world' standards from being published. This, in turn, would help the profession of singing teachers a great deal, as we rely upon research information when working with students. The Voice Foundation can serve us in the upcoming decades by setting standards for acoustic examples.

I. Titze, PhD: The Voice Foundation has become a regular place to present one's recent data – a lot of people use it as a place to go with their students so they can present up-to-date findings. There is always a steady mix of ENTs, scientists, SLPs and pedagogues, and the meeting has a high reputation, but the heated arguments have subsided.

What is hard to secure these days for beginning scientists is seed money. In Jim Gould's days, there were more donations from wealthy people. As a result, start-up grants of $5,000–30,000 were always available from TVF. Now that the voice field is growing, the amount of money per new investigator has been shrinking. There are many gifted otolaryngologists and scientists, so the money that's out there from private donors is more thinly spread.

M. Benninger, MD: Serving as Director of the Scientific Advisory Board was kind of a bittersweet thing. It was great to be able to get these remarkable people together and talk about opportunities to advance The Voice Foundation, and advance voice care, and all of those things that go with it. So it really was, in many ways, an eye-opener and a learning experience for me. I think the difficulty for us is money. So many of the things that we would have liked to be able to do through the Advisory Board, and the Scientific Advisory Board before that, we didn't have enough resources to support them. There are terrific, brilliant people with great interest, and we get together for this fabulous, collaborative meeting each year, where we share ideas and visions; but activities in The Voice Foundation revolve primarily around the Symposia and the journal. To get people to do things was difficult, because they were already very strongly invested in their other certification organizations that function year-round.

My concern, going forward, is that there are more and more competing organizations and conferences. The Voice Foundation and the *Journal of Voice* are perceived to be synonymous, and in many ways the journal helps continue to keep The Voice Foundation different from all those other organizations and meetings. Also, the voice scientists are a bigger part of The Voice Foundation symposia than any other meeting, and it is where they get to interact with clinicians.

The other meetings that have basically mimicked The Voice Foundation tend not to include the voice scientists, and have little contribution from the music education community. TVF's multidisciplinary interaction is what, to me, makes it unique. We all get to learn from experts in areas other than our own, and these are the courses and lectures where I tend to learn a lot more than I do from the medical side.

I think my concern going into the future, is succession planning. The Voice Foundation has largely been through the efforts of two brave men, Jim and Bob. When Jim died rather suddenly, Bob had already been given the leadership role. I don't think we've planned very well for the legacy of The Voice Foundation beyond Bob Sataloff, and the future may well lie in who that next generation of Voice Foundation champions are. That's my one concern moving forward.

I want to recognize the remarkable contributions of Bob and Jim, along with the other greats like Moore and Miller, and all those people like Sundberg, Titze, Baken, and Bless, to name only a few. These people, that were so passionate and supportive of this interdisciplinary approach to the care of the voice, need to be recognized.

C. Sapienza, PhD: I have high opinions of Dr Sataloff and the team of people that he has always put together. It is a mainstay and they should always be recognized for their contributions.

TVF is historic. It has always been considered to be the premier program – same time of year, same place, same 'bat-channel.' You want to encourage people to recognize that history. And I think, sometimes, you have to remind the newcomers what that history was. I'd like to see a gentle reminder of what that history was – almost like a flashback. Even if it's brief, just walking the newcomers through some of the history would be awesome.

Into the future, The Voice Foundation should be challenging those who are accepted for presentation, to be asking those novel questions, and really encouraging the innovators.

I'd like to see a focus on the business side of

practice and implementation; on what is the most cost-effective options for our patients; do we all need to have sophisticated instrumentations in our clinic? (No); and what are the tools that can be utilized, in a portable way, for us to be able to document our patients' function?

Let's integrate these fields into our discussion. Let's talk about other practicing fields that have the same type of clinical accreditation standards, and the same type of knowledge and skills that have to be obtained. I'd like to see more integration with other applied health specialists, a little bit more discussion of economics and healthcare, and we can do that within the area of voice rehab. We've done it well in the area of performance, let's continue to do that, but involve other fields as well, that may interface or interplay with us as practicing clinicians.

Patients nowadays have to have things that are really real and very pragmatic for them, and cost effective; and I think we're getting there with some of the health models and coming up, with some of the mechanisms for treatment. I'd like to hear more about those programs. Clinicians are coming because they want implementation along with theory.

R.C. Scherer, PhD: The Symposium is one of the most important functions of The Voice Foundation. Although we need smaller, focused meetings relative to narrower subfields, there is a critical place for The Voice Foundation Symposia, and that is to bring all of the voice disciplines together to share current information with each other. It fosters cross-disciplinary understanding, collaboration, deeper thinking about one's own questions, and long-term friendships that stimulate future harmony within the professions.

We have a perspective of what the other meetings do, and what keeps the Symposia quite special. But how do you satisfy all the voice professions in a limited amount of time? The Symposia have been amazing in dealing with that, but it always remains a primary question. One area that needs to be addressed is, how to attract and please students of all the voice professions? We need to make sure that they receive a great deal of satisfaction when they are at these meetings, and come away from the Symposium with something that has changed their lives.

But the role of the Symposia, the interdisciplinary aspect of The Voice Foundation, and its central mission of education and promotion and dissemination of research, are still there, alive and well. We just have to make sure that they remain quite strong and relevant.

11

Balance of Culture and Science

> Voice is the one door that takes you to the arts and takes you to medicine. I went to voice because it was the one possibility of making me balance culture and science.
>
> M. Behlau, PhD

J. LoVetri: There were very heated discussions between the PhD doctors and the MD doctors. There were all kinds of arguments about everything, and sometimes it was like a tennis match watching the arguments! There was a lot of discord between the scientists and the singing teachers. Many of the singing teachers, believed the scientists didn't have any idea how we sing or what singing teachers do, and they looked at science as a kind of affront to them. The attitude seemed to be, "You people need to know what we do, but we don't need to know what you do because what you do isn't art."

Because of all I was learning, I became a very enthusiastic supporter of The Voice Foundation and all the work that it does. I saw how important it was and, in masterclasses I taught, I would say, "You cannot be a twentieth-century singing teacher if you don't know voice science." Thirty years ago, when I presented at the New York Singing Teachers' Association, I stated to everyone, "The profession is going to go in the direction of voice science. If you don't know it now, you're going to need to know it in the future. This is not a maybe. This is a definite. Please listen to me. We are not going backward. You must know voice science." There were a lot of people in the room whose response was, "We are singing teachers, we don't need that stuff. We're artists and we understand the mystery of singing."

Through the Symposia, I finally became very comfortable with both the medical and clinical science of vocal production.

Sometimes the fur would fly at the Symposia, but gradually as the younger singing teachers came in, some of that argument diminished. There were more teachers who came from the worlds of musical theater and commercial music, who were open-minded about discourse and who truly respected the scientists, (perhaps, because many of the scientists sang, and sang well). Some of the rancor diminished and it was very nice to see that the voice teachers were more open to accepting the information – even if they didn't exactly understand immediately what to do with it.

Dr Sataloff and Dr Titze started to write for the *NATS Journal of Singing*, which helped, and Symposia participants who taught masterclasses began to integrate this voice science information into their work with singers and teachers in a way that was compatible with what they already knew. That also softened some of the discord. Of course, there will always be disagreements, but the level of anger continues to come down.

It is interesting that elite singers, who are responsible for absolute precision in their languages, musicianship, memorization, technical abilities and physicality on stage, often carry a distrust of that precision when applied to their actual vocal instrument. Rather like a formula race car driver superstitiously refusing to know how the engine works. However, once they and their pedagogues realize the value of this wealth of investigated knowledge, they become hungry for new information.

K. Ardo: I would go each year with an open mind and try to pick up new information that I could apply within my teaching, not only for singers, but for speakers and anyone that is a professional voice user. And I think it's very important for a voice teacher to be open. I have found many times that, especially with older NATS members, each person is set in their ways of teaching and they believe that how they are teaching is the correct and right way. It might be the correct and right way, but there are so many semantics and so many ways of saying that 'right way' to that particular person. One should be open to these semantics and open to understanding why, perhaps, adding this onto your knowledge might assist you and your students. That was one of the greatest gifts for me from The Voice Foundation Symposia, to have a totally open mind and be able to absorb all of the different versions of the same thing.

J. Sundberg, PhD: I think that the exchange of experiences between colleagues and young singing teachers is greatly facilitated if you have the same terminology, and if that terminology is based on tangible facts. Then you could share your experiences. If you just have your own terminology, it is like the situation in the old days where there were churches, there were religions: "I am a believer in this pedagogy, and the other ones are wrong and I'm right." It was the only way in the old days.

We talked about real-time feedback and the possibilities to combine lectures with workshops. It is quite interesting and quite encouraging to see the fascination and the great burning interest for voice function of young people who want to educate themselves to be singing teachers.

William Vennard was a key person in the development of the theoretical and practical competence of singing teachers in the US. He wrote the book, *Singing: The Mechanism and the Technique*, and I think that has raised the competence of US singing teachers much above what you see in many European countries, where many singing teachers are still deep into voodoo.

When I was younger, I often met a rather suspicious attitude in people of "Don't come and teach me, because I know already how things work." That has changed, and being an old member in the game is also helpful, actually, because people have met me, or seen me, or heard about me, and then it is much easier to ask singers to be subjects in research projects.

When I made the first attempts in synthesizing a singing voice, there was a reaction of, "Are you going to replace us with machines?" That, of course, will never happen because artistry is the essence of music in singing and in instrumental music, and that could never be replaced by machines.

K. Ardo: I had a very hard time, when I was putting together the first meetings in Canada, to have NATS teachers come. That has just changed because NATS itself has been more open to the science of voice and to understanding the science of voice. And I think that establishing the Van Lawrence Fellowship was a great idea from Dr Van Lawrence, because it got teachers to be more interested in the science and research of voice. That was a really big step. The open-mindedness, really opening your mind to all of the semantics of being able to say the same thing, but perhaps a little differently, and understanding each other's semantics.

To have all these researchers on the one side, and you have the singing teachers there, the singers and the actors, and I think that this is a wonderful thing, because each of these segments of the population of voice users and voice caregivers, their minds work in different ways. A researcher's mind works in a different way and a teacher's mind works in a different way. My mind works in a different way because I have this very perceptual muscle memory of myself and also others. But that's what makes it so interesting. That a room full of so many different ways of perceiving things and, yet, coming to the same realization right at the end of the day.

What is often surprising to the vocal pedagogues and performers who attend TVF Symposia, is the level of musicianship and talent among the scientists, doctors, and clinicians. These are people who truly love, and are fascinated by the voice. Investigating what is behind the wizard's curtain has answered some questions, while prompting many more, and does not seem to have diminished the enduring mystique around breath, phonation and artistry.

J. Sundberg, PhD: The pipe organ is a remarkable instrument. I've been interested in musical performance during my research years, and with the organ you can't do very much. You can just decide if a pipe should be silent, or if it should sound. And even with this very severe restriction of what you can do as a player, it is a very expressive and interesting instrument if it is played well. So that shows that the timetable of what is happening in music – when the tone starts and if there is a hold between them and when the following tone starts – that is an exceedingly basic and important dimension of music performance. If you only have that, you could make music; and if you don't have command over the timetable of the tones, then you are not doing any music anymore.

This is what we have in computer-played music which exactly converts the nominal durations in the score to sound. And that sounds so pathologic, which is really quite interesting. The duration and what happens in the tones is the interesting thing in music communication. With the voice you could do a continuously growing sound level and you could decrease it in a meaningful way and then you also have the possibilities to vary what the vocal folds are doing for you, so you could color the voice and make it darker or brighter. You have a lot of possibilities to continuously vary the tone quality. And that, of course, is an important set of possibilities that singers are required to use in a meaningful way. And if it is not meaningful, it's just bad singing.

You need to have a perfect command over your voice, and then you need to understand the music so that you make meaningful things with the voice as the notes and the chords and the tempos shift in the musical structure.

I. Titze, PhD: Now I am interested in looking into different vocal styles, like belt, jazz, pop, and how they can be sorted out. How do the styles differ with regard to mouth and tongue shape, and how does vocal tract shape go together with the sound that's produced? Why is Idina Menzel's mouth so wide open – is it just to show a good set of teeth, or is it an acoustic requirement? Using computer simulation, we can study styles acoustically, and how they are produced physiologically.

M. Behlau, PhD: First, I was enrolled in audiology. And then I said, well, but you know this voice area is an area that combines science, health, and culture and I was always very cultural-oriented. I always liked this kind of opening of your views through culture, and I think that the voice does that and The Voice Foundation is unique in opening the health vision.

Health professionals' vision can be very narrow because we have no time to study and read anything but our field. So we happen to be very boring, monotonous, and usually non-interesting persons. From the field of communication sciences and disorders, and the whole of otolaryngology, voice is the one door that takes you to the arts and takes you to medicine. So I felt this might be a good combination. I went to voice because it was the one possibility of making me balance culture and science.

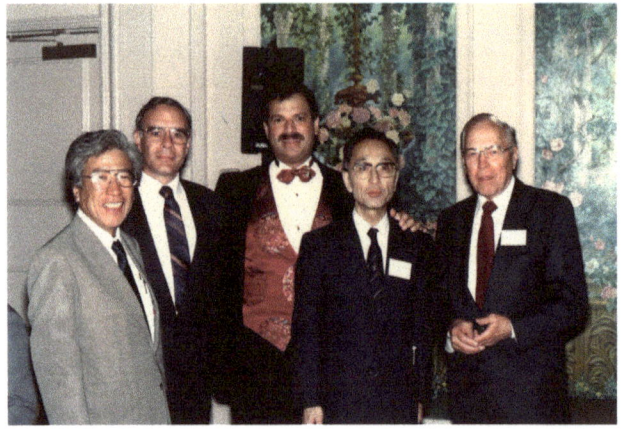

Shigeru Hirano, Ron Baken, Robert T. Sataloff, Kenzo Ishizaka, G. Paul Moore

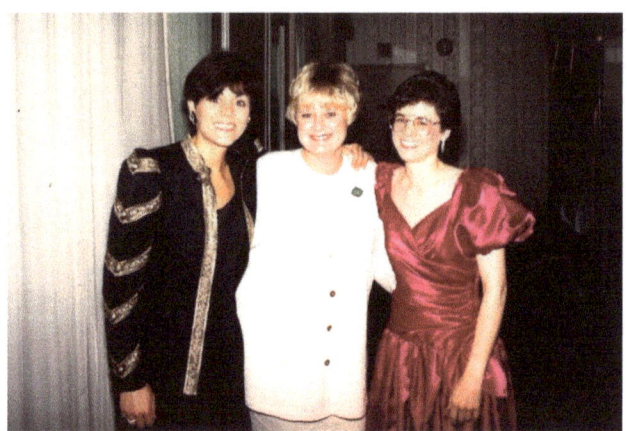

Margaret 'Peggy' Baroody, Mary Hawkshaw, Cheryl Parnell

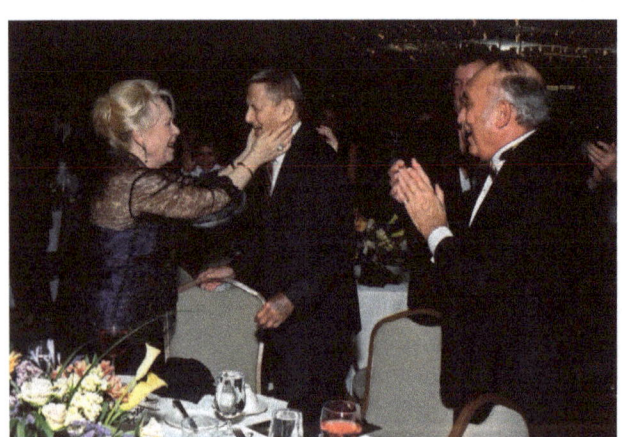

Renata Scotto, Tony Randall, Leon Fassler

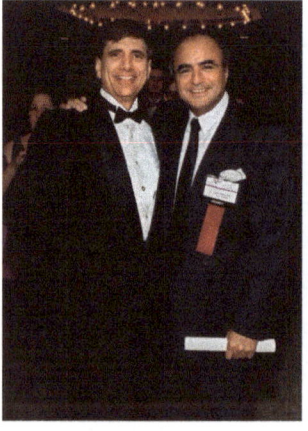

Nick Maragos, Jean Abitbol

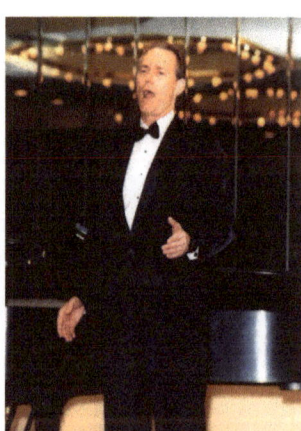

Ron Scherer

BALANCE OF CULTURE AND SCIENCE

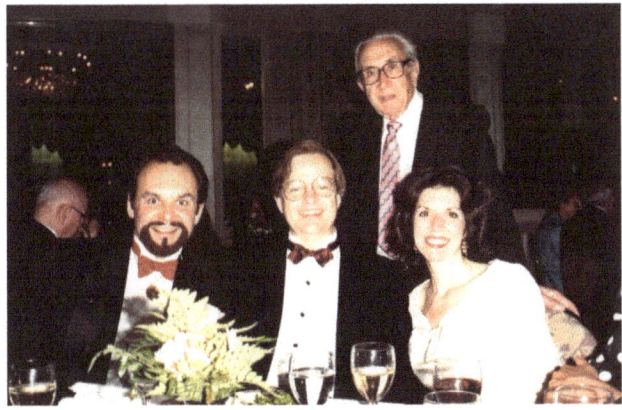

Gregory Gallivan, William Riley, Wilbur James Gould, Linda Carroll

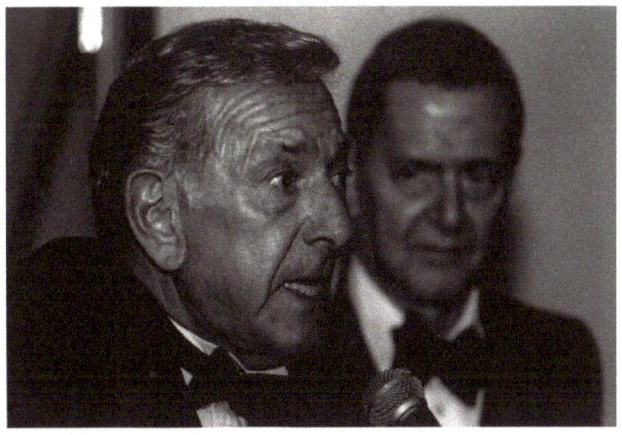

Jack Klugman, Tony Randall

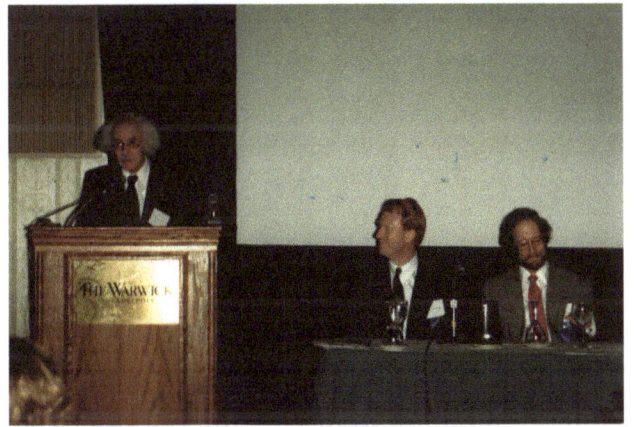

Hans von Leden, Michael Benninger, John Rubin

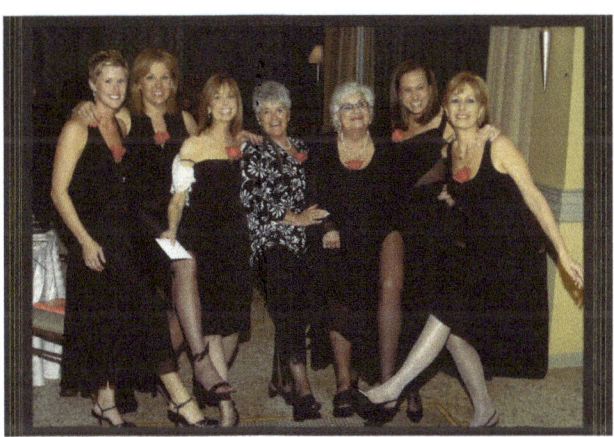

Ashley Paseman Kelley, Lorraine Ramig, Joan Lader,
Fran Lowery-Romero, Janina Casper, Gwen Korovin, Mara Behlau

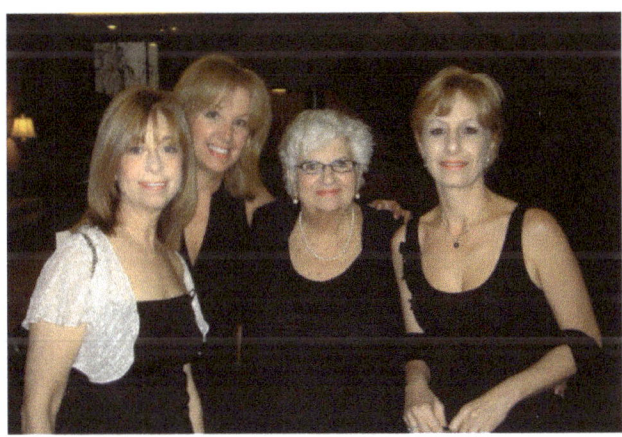

Joan Lader, Lori Ramig, Janina Casper, Mara Behlau

Mike Benninger, Leon Fassler, Shirley Verrett, George Shirley

Robert T. Sataloff, Martina Arroyo, Ben Vereen, Richard Miller, Michael Benninger

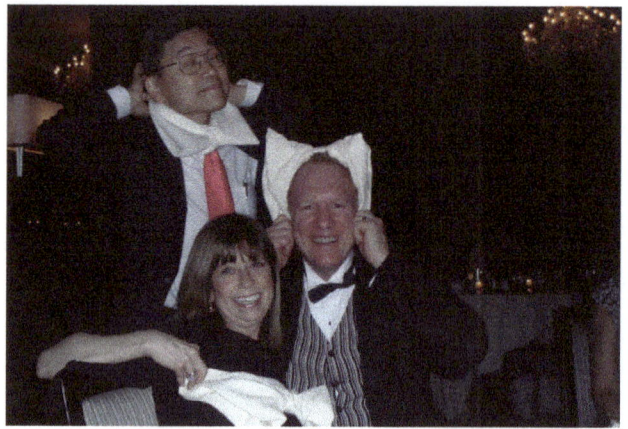
Peak Woo, Joan Lader, Michael Benninger (the famous napkin tricks)

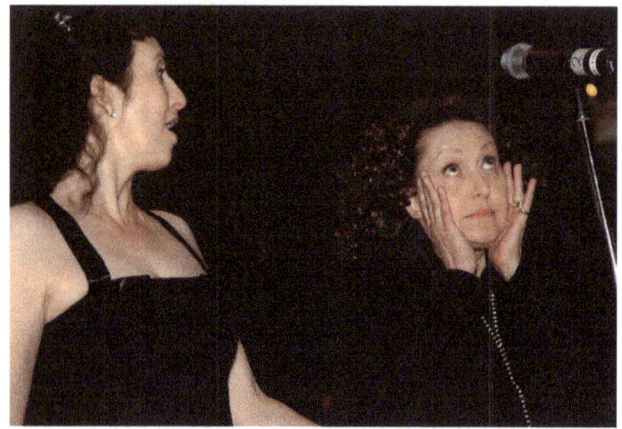
Lisa Popeil, Jeannette LoVetri

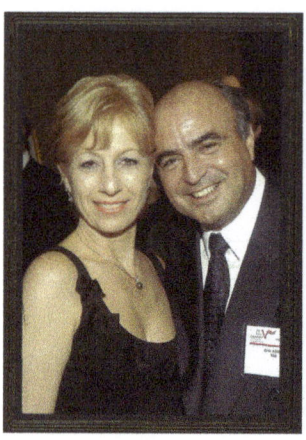
Mara Behlau, Jean Abitbol

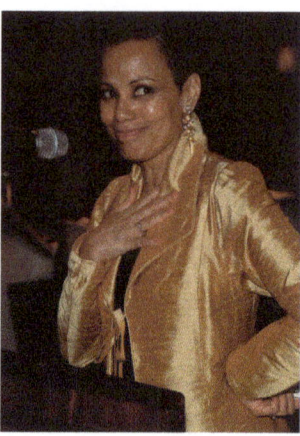
Harolyn Blackwell

Back-Stories: *Johan Sundberg, Raymond H. Colton, Harvey M. Tucker, Ronald C. Scherer*

Johan Sundberg, PhD

Head of Research Group for Music Acoustics 1970 onward, Personal Chair in Music Acoustics 1979 onward, retired 2001: KTH – Royal Institute of Technology, Stockholm
Visiting Professor: University of London
Founding Member: World Voice Consortium

When I was sixteen or seventeen, I decided to go to an organ concert on a Saturday evening, just for fun. I detected a classmate at the same concert that I had never spoken with before. We, of course, spoke a bit and became friends, and then we decided that we should build an organ together. And so we started that project and that was a very difficult project. We tried to make and made magnets, electrical magnets . . . that was a terrible thing. And then I carried on and he pulled out after a year or two, and I started to build organ pipes, wooden organ pipes.

In the end, I was arranging an inauguration concert when I had finished school, and so the bellow was under the bed, the vacuum cleaner was a fan, and I bought an old wind chest that had been in a vault. The tracker action came out in the short side, not on the long side of the wind chest but it came out the wrong way, so I got the bass up here and the treble down there. It was very bad luck, but I solved the problem. The organ still sits, like a silent elephant, in the bedroom.

I was very fascinated by organ music, and I still am. So I made up my doctoral dissertation about the acoustics of organ pipes. Then I came into contact with Gunnar Fant and his lab, and had a wonderful mentor, Frans Fransson, who helped me with doing the measurements and understanding them. I had a lot of friends here at the Speech Transmission laboratory at KTH, which was the name of the department in those days.

My experience of singing was a more natural connection to the department. When I had finished my doctoral dissertation in 1966, I applied for a grant on the voice and got it from 1967, or 1968. That started my research on the singing voice and it was carried out at the same department. So that was the transition from organ pipes to human pipes.

When I came to Uppsala for my musicology studies, I was asking the organ player in the cathedral there if I could practice on one of the organs. "Well that won't work," he said, "because I have so many services here." But he said I could sing in the choir. I had never sung before then, and I didn't dare to say that I had never sung, so I went to the choir rehearsals and tried.

Then I took the lower education track for organists that required singing lessons, and I went to a crazy lady there in Uppsala, which was very interesting. The social ties that were offered in the choral society were a significant complementation of my life so I got very interested in singing as well. And that was another reason why I started with singing research.

A quarter century later, there was a celebration with the choir and I was sitting next to one of the sopranos and she asked, "When did you start singing in choirs?" and I said it was 1955, and she said, "I was two years old then." That was sort of thought-provoking, and I decided maybe I should do something else. I started to sing Lieder with an accompanist and found that very interesting and challenging. The need for expressivity is much more severe when you alone and are responsible for what happens in the music, than if you're in a chorus ensemble where your neighbors and the conductor are deciding what should happen.

That was providing a sort of in-depth contact with the lyrics, the music and harmony, and the questions of: Why this piece was composed in this way? What happened with the emotional ambience at this point in the composition? And, what then happened in the composition? I think such things are very, very fascinating. After my musicological studies, I studied with a lovely singing teacher who had a very profound interest in expressivity, meaningfulness, and lyrics, and that was also stimulating. That was the reason I decided that I should have a debut concert on my fiftieth birthday in a public concert hall. It was a great experience to sing, not only with an accompanist, but also with an audience in front of you.

Raymond H. Colton, PhD

Emeritus Professor: Communication Sciences and Disorders, Syracuse University

In college my major was in social studies and history, with a minor in speech and drama, but when I went to graduate school at the University of Connecticut, I majored in speech pathology. While I was studying my Masters, I had several courses in science that had to do with the voice. I became interested in the scientific aspect of speech, so when I decided to go for the PhD, there were only a couple of schools that focused on the voice, and I ended up at the University of Florida. So it was a circuitous route, but I got there. In the early 1970s, I was involved in community theatre, in plays, comedies, and musicals, and I am still interested in history, and am reading it more now that I am retired.

My University of Connecticut professor, Harry Cooker, who was very much interested in voice – especially breathing – influenced my path. My first, and longtime teaching job was at Upstate Medical Center (now Upstate Medical University). I obtained a position in the Department of Otolaryngology and Communication Sciences, where I focused mostly on research. I was part of a good research group within the department and stayed for twenty-five years. I became more into the medical aspects of speech and voice, as I worked closely with physicians and other healthcare workers.

My dissertation was on Vocal Registers, where the vocal folds go into a switching mechanism as you go into a higher pitch, and I was looking at some of the acoustic characteristics of the modal and falsetto registers. Registers, of course, are big in the singing world. The singers and singing teachers had different names than we did, but we soon became clear to each other as to what we meant.

I became involved with singers very early in the studies for the PhD. Harry had me contact the Chair of the Music department and they were very cooperative in helping me with my research. The Chair of the department was a member of my committee, so we used singers and agreed as to what the registers were.

Harvey M. Tucker, MD, FACS

Otolaryngology
University Hospitals Case Medical Center
Professor of Otolaryngology–Head and Neck Surgery: Case Western Reserve University School of Medicine

I grew up in Philadelphia and my father was a jeweler – although, actually a licensed pharmacist, then a research pharmacist. We're Jewish, and at Christmas and other Christian holidays my father would volunteer to be the pharmacist in the local Catholic hospital so that the people there could take time off. So I grew up thinking that if you can do something that is helpful to your fellow man, that's what you do.

I wanted to be a veterinarian. As the time approached for me to actually make a decision about what to do next, I was under pressure from one of the professors there to go on in zoology and become a PhD in zoology, and from my mother, who kindly would say, "Look if you're going to take the trouble to go to medical school, you might as well take care of people." Well, that's true.

It was the time of Vietnam, and the Philadelphia Naval Hospital at the time was a very large, a very excellent facility, so I chose the Navy. They would provide summer clerkships with pay for up to sixty days every time you got a vacation, which looked really good because I was married and had no other income.

I wanted to work in surgery, but was told that my best bet was to apply for one of the minor surgical specialties. And, as it happened, they had a full residency in ENT available. During this sixty day period I was the only clinical clerk, and the residents were very nice, so I even got to do certain minor surgical procedures and take care of patients I would not have even seen before my junior, or senior year of medical school. That's how I decided ENT was the right profession.

Ronald C. Scherer, PhD

Distinguished Research Professor: Department of Communication Sciences and Disorders, Bowling Green State University, Ohio

Like many other people associated with The Voice Foundation, I have always been interested in many different concepts, disciplines, and applications – from sciences, through the arts. I was always interested in mathematics and music so I grew up doing well in mathematics, and always played an instrument or two and enjoyed singing.

My instruments were primarily French horn, some piano, and a little bit of a few others. I got pretty good as a French hornist, but when I got to college, the orchestra played at the same time as the men's glee club. I had to make a choice, and I went to the glee club. I graduated with a bachelor's degree in mathematics, then I started over as a sophomore in music at Indiana University. I had wanted to be a singer ever since I heard Jerome Hines sing, and I wanted to do what he did.

But then after a year and a half at IU, having great experiences in vocal pedagogy with Ralph Appleman, I decided to go into speech and hearing and subsequently received a master's in Speech Pathology and Audiology. Throughout this time I was very interested in the voice, and decided to go on for a doctorate in voice research. I was fortunate to get accepted at the University of Iowa with James Curtis as my advisor. He knew I was into math and all that, and asked if I had read this article by van den Berg on flow resistance in a larynx model. Curtis handed it to me and, basically, I couldn't understand a word in it.

So I continued to deal with that, took some engineering courses, and built wax models of the larynx and cast them and, eventually, that turned out to be part of my dissertation. What was truly wonderful was that Ingo Titze came to replace James Curtis, who was retiring, and that was a most fortuitous thing for me. We started working together and connected through my dissertation.

At my first Symposium at Juilliard, I gave a talk on van den Berg's equation and the modeling work. Bob Sataloff very graciously likes to tell people that nobody understood my talk, "but look how far he's come now." It is a great compliment, and I appreciate it.

12

Seeing Sound

> We may be sorry that we didn't keep the original analog signals, because they contain more information and different information than we have in the digitized acoustical signal.
>
> R. T. Sataloff, MD, DMA

The capturing and measuring of sound spectra has evolved from the early days of projecting the frequencies against a wall, or pressing your own record to play while spinning the phonellograph in a dark room:

R. C. Scherer, PhD: Minoru Hirano visited the University of Iowa to do some training and research in electromyography, and the EMG was recorded on a strip chart recorder – a recorder that has a page coming out, and a pen writing the signal on the paper. He would lay that piece of paper out and, with a ruler, mark what he thought was the average or RMS [root mean square current, or voltage] through the signal. Then he would estimate that average value, and his data would be not just analog, but highly subjective in this quasi-objective way. And he would report his visual measures of the EMG across these different conditions. It was brilliant.

R. H. Colton, PhD: Some of the machines we used at Florida were pretty old. We did not have much in the way of computer facilities then. One machine we used during our training was a phonellograph. It was very simple, consisting of a large, circular drum, around which you placed a piece of photo-sensitive paper. A bright light was focused onto the paper. The light was modulated with the acoustic signal you wanted to analyze, and you could see the waveform. One point: this analysis had to be conducted in the dark. When developed, the paper would show the sound oscillations, from which you could measure fundamental frequency.

With computers, you could do a lot more in the way of acoustic analysis. We used reel-to-reel tapes to record the sound samples, but the medium quickly changed to cassette tape and then went straight to digital. It meant that we could process a lot more information within a certain period of time, and we could look at different aspects of voice. More sophisticated techniques of analysis began to come out and then we could analyze sound in much more sophisticated ways.

The spectrograph is an analog device to look at a spectrum; the frequency composition of a sound.

It puts the results of its analysis on heat sensitive paper: the stronger the sound, the stronger the burn. Developed during WW2, they probably started making them in the late 1940s, and they were used to look at speech. It was limited as to the strength of sound it could portray, but was good for speech purposes. We used it a lot in the 1950s for analyzing speech and vowels. A lot of good work came from using that technique.

You had to have a breathing device because it was pretty smoky in the room from all the burning paper. We did that a lot with cancer patients. If we had had the digital earlier, we wouldn't have had to burn so much paper!

J. Sundberg, PhD: The evolution and development of voice science has been immense. I think that the general awareness of voice production has been developing greatly over the last decades and I just checked in *Journal of Voice*, *Folia Phoniatrica*, and *Logopedics, Phonatrics, Vocology* and summed the articles that have been dealing with singing in one way or the other, and that was up to six hundred or so.

The technical means to do research are huge today. With Excel sheets you can fill an entire sheet with equations and numbers and you can increase the number of subjects and you can increase the number of conditions, so it is quite a nice situation today, as compared with before.

One thing that has been very important in the understanding of the voice, and of the singing voice in particular, is that we have possibilities to measure sub-glottic pressure without putting balloons or making holes in people, like they did in the seventies. And you can peel off the contributions to the sound radiated from the lip opening by inverse filtering. Inverse filtering was a hell before, taking lots of time, and you got one or two flow glottograms showing what the voice source looked like under certain conditions, but now it is no problem to get hundreds of them.

You can keep track of what the filtering is doing, and you get statistics showing you how the voice source is affected by changes of sub-glottal pressure, glottal adduction and pitch, these three continuously variable voice control parameters. We could measure pitch and we could measure sub-glottal pressure as the oral pressure during 'p' occlusion, and that means that we could plot glottogram parameters as a function of sub-glottal pressure at different pitches, and see what the glottal adduction is doing. This has been an enormously important increase of the possibilities to analyze the voice.

If you just take the radiated sound, you don't know who produced the things that you measure and it is just a spectrum or a waveform, but if you peel off what the formants did, then you can study the voice source in isolation and relate it to the control parameters sub-glottal pressure and pitch. Then you can describe different vocal styles in a much more meaningful and instructed way than before, when you just looked at, perhaps, the electroglottogram and the radiated sound.

J Sundberg, PhD: Is the formant the spectral peak or the resonance? For me, formant is nothing but vocal tract resonance. Resonance in the vocal tract; that's a formant.

And then things come rather easy, because you could control the frequencies of the formants by articulation, otherwise you have a lot of factors that affect the frequencies of the formants. That will be a terrible swampland if you say that a formant is a spectrum peak. Imagine that you have a high soprano singing at 1,000 Hz, and then she has one partial at each 1,000 Hz. So then if you should keep the idea that a formant is a spectrum peak, then she has one spectrum peak per partial, and she can't really do very much about it, and it's not related to vowel quality either. So I feel that it is confusing to mix up spectrum peak and formants. They should be kept apart and a formant is a resonance in the vocal tract.

R. H. Colton, PhD: The switch to digital was probably in the early 1970s. It was done before, but my first computer analysis was done on bigger computers, difficult to get in and out of. The first mini-computers were basic and didn't have the capacity to do the kind of work we wanted in the beginning, and it took a while for them to develop. By the late 1980s and 1990s, they started to come into their own and have gotten better since then.

With the techniques we had, we were limited as to what kinds of measurements we could get. We could analyze fundamental frequency, the amplitude or the strength of the sound, we could actually get what they call perturbation, or the variation in the frequency, from the analog signal, but it is much easier in a digital world to do that. You can basically identify the period of the sound, then just let the computer go through and find the other periods. You used to have to do that by hand. And with the computers, it is much faster and many times much more accurate too, as they can get down to very small periods of time, which you really couldn't do on a piece of paper because the width of the pencil you used would permit how accurate you could be. Even with a very thin, sharp pencil.

J. Sundberg, PhD: Yeah, the switch to digital was a great relief. When you went to do lectures, I had, I don't know how many kilos of equipment in the trunk, and had to drag it in airplanes and, oi-oi-oi, that was terrible. And slow. When you had to make tape loops and that was terrible. If you wanted to make a spectrum analysis, you needed to make a tape loop with a sustained vowel, and then let it run revolution, after revolution, after revolution, after revolution on a tape recorder while analyzing it. It was a wet blanket over research.

Then, to write, in the old days, with the electrical typewriters – and then you saw that in the ten pages of the stencil there was a mistake in the first page. You didn't want to go to the secretary and ask her to rewrite ten pages, but she could correct the error page by a sort of paint. But she didn't want to paint over the entire paragraph, just one line was the upper limit, so you needed to change the text so that the number of characters was the same but there was no mistake in it. The space was limited to what it was before, and you had to squeeze your truth into that. It was quite an exercise for writing.

Now, when you see how you do the writing with moving sentences upstairs and downstairs, it is so simple. That was 1980, and I was on my way to Sydney then. There was an acoustic conference there, I think, and I went with Jan Gauffin, who was my co-author in many articles. He was also a computer activist, and he came there with a brand new computer that had Wordstar. You didn't need to do the erasing – that was such a relief – and things went so quickly. So, digitalization has been a revolution in research, both for writing and for processing data. That is for sure.

And then also, of course, the possibilities to do synthesis. You measure and measure and measure, and then you find some things that seem to be typical of what you measure and then you want to find out if this is the entire story, or did I miss some important aspects? Then you can plug in your measured characteristics into the synthesizer and listen to what it sounds like. It is merciless in revealing what you forgot. But it is also pointing towards where you should go.

And I know that many European voice teachers use voice synthesizers, like the Madde synthesizer, quite a bit in their teaching to show effects that they found interesting, such as vibrato rate and vibrato extent, the speed of vibrato, and the width of the vibrato. That's so easy to demonstrate with this synthesizer. And the singer's formant cluster also; just bring the higher formants close together and everybody could hear it. And, today, you can look at the synthesized tone in real time. You can listen to it and see it on the screen, and that makes it so tangible. Then you can point with your finger – this is the singer's formant cluster, and listen to it. Such things are entirely different now than they used to be when we had a big cabinet of things, and fifty knobs to turn, and if one was wrong it wouldn't show anything. Terrible, yes.

R. C. Scherer, PhD: When we started the Recording and Research Center at the Denver Center for the Performing Arts in 1983, we purchased probably the best A to D converter with multiple channels for speech research, and it cost, like, sixty thousand dollars at that time for eight channels. Plus, computers at that time were pretty stingy. Our computer manager gave us 1,500 KB and told us not to go over that, and we always complained about not having enough space to do anything.

But that was what it was like in the early 1980s. It was very expensive to buy computers. It was very expensive to buy any A to D converters that were any good with AC and DC coupling, mind you, and we almost had no space on a computer to do anything. Now, of course, the A to D converters that we use are really fine, better, and a lot less expensive And, obviously, computers hold a lot more memory. From a research point of view, that's one of the biggest differences between then and now.

M. Benninger, MD: It made it easier to record, measure and exchange information, and we can apply some objectivity to some of the things that we are hearing, that would be hard to do in analog. I will tell you that it hasn't completely converted. We have a full recording studio in our clinic, and the sound gurus have told us that there are still some things that are recorded in analog and then converted. I don't know that, from a voice physician standpoint, it really mattered to us one way or the other, other than the simplicity of how we could do things and exchange information.

From a qualitative standpoint do I think they're dramatically different? I happen to like the sound of vinyl records.

R. C. Scherer, PhD: We still use analog equipment, of course. When you have a box and you give it a stimulus, like some sort of pressure or something, you still get a voltage out. The digital aspect is what comes after that. It's what you do with those signals – you digitize them into computer files.

R. T. Sataloff, MD, DMA: *Did the move from analog to digital affect your work?*

In some ways favorably, and in some ways unfavorably. I hold a minority opinion in this. Most people feel that digital acoustic signals are a great improvement. At the present time, they probably are; however, digital signals are compressed and manipulated. That means that some of the original data are lost. Right now, our analysis equipment is so insensitive that that doesn't mean anything; however, if we are ever successful in developing much more sophisticated analytical equipment, we may be sorry that we didn't keep the original analog signals, because they actually contain more information and different information than we have in the digitized acoustical signal, and I am hopeful that someday our analysis ability will be good enough that we may want the rest of the signal when we reanalyze old samples. That is a minority opinion.

C. Sapienza, PhD: With the change to digital, data analysis is easier and more available; they've automated things, your filters and input are digital. You can crop and clean and filter and maneuver and manipulate and generate lots of programs and algorithms to do measurements. You know it's no different from when your Father said, "I used to walk three miles to…" I think you can self-teach better than you were able to do in the past, where you needed a little bit more hands-on training. I think it is easier to teach the students. It's simplified.

In some ways the basis of it hasn't really changed. The methodology is similar, but the tools have become smaller and finer in their measurements, and you don't have to make as many choices. You can be a little more discriminate in the tools that you want to use to get the outcome that you are trying to achieve. I mean just look at stroboscopy. Paul Moore in the early 1980s, and even when I was there in the early 1990s, we were doing that with analog lighting and film, rows and rows, and miles of film. So, it's changed tremendously.

13

Greater Resolution and Precision

I would say that the science of voice has moved forward because of greater resolution in time, greater resolution in space (whether that space is outside the tissue or inside the tissue), and greater precision in surgical procedures. Those are great advancements, plus the improved training of practitioners in the various disciplines of voice.

R. Scherer, PhD

M. Behlau, PhD: I believe that a good clinician needs good eyes, ears, and a good brain. This helps a lot. Of course, if you are a good clinician with good equipment, you are going to do wonders. If you are a bad clinician with good equipment, you keep on doing bad. So I believe good equipment helps only the ones who were already good without the wonderful equipment. In Brazil, we developed low-cost equipment such as acoustic programs. I developed, with a Brazilian company, more than eight software programs in acoustic analysis, more than six EBPs apps that are at the Apple store, and very low cost equipment and software.

I would adore to have Louis Vuitton handbags and to have designer clothing, but it's not my pocket, and neither is it for most of my colleagues here. I would adore to have the first-level equipment, but this is not Brazilian reality. So, what happened is that we decided to make equipment that could fit the Brazilian financial pocket. I believe that today, where everything is reduced in size and also in price, where you have portable equipment that you can perform an endoscopy with an iPhone, with a micro-camera, that we are facing changes. But still what is needed is a good eye, a good ear, and a good brain – a good mind. Equipment is wonderful, but equipment is extra.

―――――――――

H. M. Tucker, MD: Well we have now gone, almost exclusively, to flexible instruments and those are very important as they give us tremendous advantages in diagnosis, but less so in management. The flexible laryngoscope, which we all use, I use several of them every day when I see patients, they are a huge breakthrough.

Now we're using flexible nasoscopes, flexible esophoscopes, but the one drawback to them is that they do not give you much ability to manipulate things. So if you have a foreign body to take care of, which we often have to take care of, it's much easier to manage that with the rigid instrumentation. The problem is, in order to use the rigid instrumentation, you have to have a lot of experience. The residents that are coming up today are all trained to use those instruments but they don't see anywhere near the numbers of patients that require it, that we used to see during my residency training and during the early years of my practice. But the flexible instrumentation has been a huge advantage, and the other really big advantage of course has been the laser.

I was involved in the development of the laser. I had the first commercial laser in the United States from Sharp I.M., here in the Cleveland Clinic, which is where I was after I left Syracuse. Model 0002. I don't think it's still being used, but we have it. And I was involved in some of the early work in using the laser in the larynx. Those two were the biggest breakthroughs.

R.C. Scherer, PhD: Now, you can record more signals during voice and speech production and better determine the relationships of the production variables. So there's a deeper understanding of the body's use in making sounds.

Before, you might study pitch, you might study some more isolated variable. I would say one of the more important aspects of progress in our field was in the 1970's, when Martin Rothenburg came up with his aerodynamic mask system. His system is one of the most important in the world for voice research. You can estimate pressures and measure flows and then, with other noninvasive devices, get a pretty good picture about how voice is being produced. This multi-signal recording and analysis is one of the more important advancements for understanding the voice and the variables that are important to controlling voice production.

For research and for science, that kind of enhancement of instrumentation – where we can look at finer detail of the time measures, of the acoustic measures, of the airflows and air pressures, where we are refining our ideas about how the voice is produced – relates directly to enhancing the training of those who have to use that information: speech and language pathologists, voice and speech scientists, voice and speech coaches, singing teachers, surgeons and physicians.

C.R. Stasney, MD: Strobes gave us the ability to communicate with other people. Some people just can't paint a word picture when they are describing lesions, and such. Doctors are terrible, and I'm indicting my whole profession, but there are very few English majors in medicine. So many scientists, when you read a scientific article (except for Sataloff) it's just, "What is he trying to say?" Using a quadruple negative to say a positive.

R.T. Sataloff, MD, DMA: *As equipment and instruments have been refined, what can be measured now or measured differently?*

Well, lots of things. First, the voice signal itself, as well as the airflow and aerodynamics of the voice. One of the reasons why voice didn't exist as an accepted specialty long before I helped get it started, was that there was no way to measure voice signals. There was no equivalent of an audiometer. Consequently people were unable to assess outcomes of treatment – medical, voice therapy, or surgery – in any kind of a rigorous fashion. Developing voice laboratories helped solve that problem for diagnostic and outcomes purposes. So, over the years we've seen lots of improvements in technology to measure the voice acoustically and in other ways.

We've also seen substantial advances in neuromuscular assessment, particularly laryngeal electromyography (EMG). When I wrote my first book on the care of the voice, electromyography got one paragraph. By the second edition it got a chapter. And now I have an entire book on the subject that's in its second edition. So, there have been huge, huge advances in that field. When I trained and when we got started, LEMG didn't exist in clinical settings, although there'd been reports of it back as far as 1944. But nobody used it. Recently, we took a look at our experience, and we've done more than eight thousand. That's a big change.

And, of course, there's strobovideolaryngoscopy and high-speed video, which allow assessment of the vibratory margin of the vocal fold much more discreetly than was possible before. So, we can see, as well as measure whether our voice results after surgery are good or bad; whether there is a mucosal wave, or whether there is scar and no mucosal wave. When I was training at the University of Michigan in the late 1970s, we couldn't do that. We'd operate, the voice would be terrible, we'd look with the mirror and the vocal folds looked straight; so we'd send patients to a psychiatrist. But now we can look and see if the vocal fold edge is moving the way it's supposed to. That was impossible before. We are pretty good at it with stroboscopy, but the worse the voice is, the less valid stroboscopy is. So, now there's practical high-speed video for the challenging cases.

K. Ardo: Well, the great understanding from being able to see what is going on and not only perceive, has been able to kindle new research as to how to deal with certain diagnoses. And to be able to do research and follow it through from the beginning; let's try this particular technique and let's see how it will be in six weeks and to be able to watch how it changes – how the acoustical measurements will change.

Also, with the different methods and techniques in speech-language pathology, you're now able to perceive and watch the differences and how quickly the edema on vocal folds will go down, by using them in a certain way, or by using certain techniques of resonance therapy, and so on. I think that it definitely has made for an understanding of how to get faster recovery with certain techniques, because research has been done for twenty, or twenty-five years now.

The era of strobovideolaryngoscopy has helped people that have dysphonias and dystonias, and you're able to pick up on different health issues a little more quickly. If someone has Parkinson's or MS, they're paying more attention to how the vocal folds are working because it is an indication you are able to recognize and perceive in order to diagnose them more thoroughly.

I don't think that twenty years ago, that person with Parkinson's would be going to an otolaryngologist to get some answers. But I definitely feel that, today, with the technology that exists and the strobovideolaryngoscopies, you're able to see how definitely something neurological was happening and be able to explain it, be able to get a diagnosis faster.

J. Sundberg, PhD: I think the digital version of inverse filtering, the DeCap software, has been opening a new era in voice research, because you could really get information on the glottal airflow, which you could control by sub-glottal pressure and glottal adduction So that is an extremely important tool for research today.

And then synthesizers should be developed. The Madde synthesizer is a vowel machine, so it is fine for synthesizing vowels, but if we had a realistic sounding synthesizer that could also produce consonants and swell tones and variations, then you could return to music performance, sung performance of music, and get reliable and important information about the essence of vocal art.

I had a fantastic experience when a thesis worker wanted to build a synthesizer, an organ, (every engineer who wanted to make a thesis in those days wanted to make an electrical organ) and Jan Gauffin convinced him to make a singing synthesizer instead. It had a wonderful voice and sounded like a fantastic baritone. After some other contributions from thesis workers, I could connect it to the computer and combine it with a text-to-speech synthesis program that two of my friends at the lab had been doing.

So we started to do score-to-singing performance and then, when I inserted phrasing rules, so that the singer was showing where the phrase boundaries were and also paying attention to the harmonic progressions in the piece, I could add piano accompaniment to the synthesized computer controlled performance and that was a breakthrough in singing synthesis, because it sounded exactly like a human being. I presented that at a symposium at IRCAM in Paris, I think in 1976, and there was spontaneous applause. They found it fantastic. It didn't have an electronic timbre accent. This MUSSE synthesizer sounded like a real man. And when he wanted to show where the phrase boundaries were, it was irresistible. It was fantastic. But now MUSSE is dead and the computer program is gone, and I haven't found or heard of any comparable singing synthesizer.

―――――――

M. Benninger, MD: With better instruments, we could measure things differently. We could measure semitones, we could measure whether or not a person could alter loudness without changing pitch, we could distinguish objectively why certain voices are better than others. Now we're starting to be able to make some determinations about fundamental genetic changes that may be related to differences in voice.

But the perception of voice has so much subjectivity that I don't know that we can make quantitative decisions about quality. In other words, if we were dealing with people who primarily treated opera singers, they wouldn't be very impressed with Rod Stewart's voice. And if you're somebody that really likes hip hop or alternative music, do you care that there is vibrato in a soprano's aria? You don't at all. So I think we can measure why voices sound the way that they sound, but I don't think we can apply culturally-based decisions related to quality onto the differences between different genres of music. Now within a genre, we probably could use those tools to measure things that would be consistent with differences in quality.

I have been visiting China and have done some distance-based consultations on a couple of very famous Chinese opera singers. When I listen to their voices I can hear these beautiful, rich voices. But when they get into the more traditional Chinese/Peking opera, there is a somewhat twangy (by western standards) Chinese presentation which I find interesting but qualitatively it is not the same as someone singing more traditional European opera, like Mozart. For me personally, I always have liked the cutting edge kind of pop/rock/alternative scene and culture and in many ways these are my preferred music style.

―――――――

J. Sundberg, PhD: So we are living in the right time. Also what has increased the possibilities for voice science these days is the possibility to analyze things in real time. It is not possible to describe a sound so that other people understand what you are talking about, because there is no terminology. What's a sharp sound? What's a dull one? That's very unclear. But now in the summer course that I've been running, I have workshops where people produce different types of sounds and look at the display to see one or two aspects of what they are doing.

One very fascinating possibility is to put the fiberscope so that you can see what the glottis is doing when you laugh and when you clear your throat and when you sing – different things. You could also do the same thing for breathing behavior. How much do you expand the ribcage? How much do you expand the abdominal wall when you inhale? And you could provide real-time feedback for the voice source if you have a mask and an inverse filter available. When you have this experience you feel how it feels to do this, you see how it looks, and you hear the sound of your voice. Then the conceptualization of the voice parameters becomes much more robust and tangible than if you are just trying to tell 'placement of the tone', a rather hazy concept, even though it may work with some, or many students in the studio. It is good to know about the reality if you should talk with colleagues.

14

Exploring Beyond Habit

It thrills me to watch the mystical aspects of singing and speech confront the definitions of science and medicine and start to meet at the edges. I don't know anyone who can better articulate and realize this synthesis than Dr Sataloff.

Maria Russo

Those who study the voice are surrounded by questions with slippery, vague, or multiple answers. The presenters at the Tenth Symposium in June 1981, raised some of the questions still being addressed in 2015, such as, What is good vocal health while aging? What is a good, supported breath? What improvements can be made in technology?

The following excerpts from the Transcript offer a small window into the era.

W.J. Gould, MD: About eleven years ago, we were sitting on the Opera steps at Barcelona, attending a meeting of voice scientists and laryngologists. To be frank, we did not know how to talk to each other. We had no common language. We had no common exchange. There were a few voice teachers, and none of us knew what the other meant when he spoke professionally. I also remember that Dr Barry Wyke spoke about 'vocal folds' and many of us wondered what he was talking about. Other things of a similar nature occurred. This small group sat on the Opera steps and said in effect, "Look, we have to learn to talk to each other." How should we go about doing it? We took our friends and gathered together and ten years ago we had about thirty-four people here, in this auditorium. It was a core group and the majority of them are still here, by the way.

Tom Shipp, at the very first session said, "I don't know what we're talking about, I only understand the larynx and I don't know about anything else." Gradually, he began to take voice lessons, acting lessons, and has learned how to be a holistic investigator with respect to voice.

This, then, is the essence of my message to you. Ten years ago we decided that we would try, and I think that within reasonable bounds, we've come close to succeeding. I hope that this message, in its very repetition, will continue in these same terms: this is a session which will enable us to cooperate and to understand each one of us from his own perspective.

Cynthia Hoffmann: The advent of the Tenth Symposium started my annual re-evaluation and mental perusal of the singing process and the role of the Symposia in the future.

I began by considering the learning process and the way it often occurs in the voice studio. There, we deal with sound, sensation, physical experience, emotion, and so on, to bring the student to his or her unique experience of those elements. The information usually has to be repeated in a variety of ways, sometimes once or twice, sometimes incessantly, year after year. We hope that, one day, the student will walk into the studio and reveal this experience or insight as if it had been newly created. And, of course, that is exactly what has happened. They usually say "I have made a discovery" and then proceed to tell you in your own words what you have been endeavoring to communicate. However, this description often returns to you transformed somewhat from the original version – it comes from the perspective of the individual.

For me, the Symposia have been doing quite the same thing. At the moment of reception, one may or may not understand or know how to use the information, but the fact that it has been presented from various perspectives creates a climate where its recreation from an individual point of view can occur.

———

Harry Hollien, PhD: After the excitement of World War II (exciting things like – What type of voice is best for aircraft communications? Is that really Hitler, or his double, making all those radio broadcasts?), we saw Voice Science quietly slipping into a scientific backwater. By then, it was agreed that the vocal folds vibrated by moving laterally then medially (or was it vice versa?) rather than fluttering alternately upward and downward as Robert West had been saying. And one of the big issues was whether or not the vocal folds became systematically longer and shorter as a function of change in vocal frequency.

As you can understand, I am happy to have been able to contribute to the solution of this latter mystery, but am a little unhappy that people never have caught on to the fact that the mechanism of vocal fold 'lengthening' isn't that at all. Rather, it is that the vocal folds are shortened for phonation – and then varied in length as a function of changing frequency.

[…] The cry became: "What is new in your research" (not what is 'good')! A Nobel Laureate had difficulty in maintaining one of his grants because he wanted to continue a highly successful line of inquiry and not start a new one. […] In those early days of the 1970s we all were discouraged. Wilbur James Gould attacked the problem! His approach was deceptively simple: (1) pursue those ideas that appeared to have merit, and (2) find other people (mostly scientists) who could keep the ideas flowing on those rare occasions when he, himself, experienced a dry spell.

[…] The concept of voice registers is hardly new; indeed it has been an issue of controversy among voice pedagogists for over 300 years. We are now beginning to understand that there are a variety of registers – some relate to speaking, some relate to singing, and others relate to both. […] It is encouraging that so many voice teachers now understand the nature of registers and can deal with them effectively. In this regard, it makes little difference if the singing teacher simply 'removes' the register, as does Beverley Johnson, modifies/adapts it, as does Ellen Faull, or actually utilizes it in teaching, as does Oren Brown.

[…] Concepts such as 'tone brilliance', 'ring', 'focus' and/or 'singer's formant' have been proposed, discussed and debated lengthily. The dimensions of the singer's formant are beginning to be understood. We are learning that this entity relates to the shape of the vocal tract, to the phonated frequency level and, especially, to the level of output energy. What is even more important, however, is that it was during this past decade that most scholars agreed to the existence of 'ring' and then began – for the first time – to attempt to determine its boundaries/dimensions and, especially, its causes/nature.

[…] More is known (by far) about our neurosensory systems than about our neuromotor systems. There are now entire laboratories which focus on the motor control of speech and voice.

[…] The advance of technology during the past decade has been spectacular; indeed the progress in computers alone is breathtaking. Yet we have not kept up! Fiberoptic approaches to laryngeal viewing still are in a primitive state: ultra high-speed laryngeal photography is about where it was in the 1940s.

[…] As of late there has been a resurgence of interest in such issues as the anatomy, morphology and histology of the larynx. Models of the larynx, especially those that explain how the vocal folds move, and under what conditions, can be very useful. The Landagraf/Flanagan two-mass models are somewhat simpler in their conception and are a little easier to understand than are the multimass models of Ingo Titze and his associates (notably Ronald Scherer). Basically, Titze attempts to build his models in such a way that they incorporate available empirical knowledge. Hence, his approximations tend to be more realistic in nature and more robust in their predictive ability. It would appear, even intuitively, that a model based on 'that which is' should be more powerful than one which is based on 'what might be' – other things being equal.

[…] One of the very real, and very welcome, changes that took place was a general shifting of interest from the pathological voice to the normal voice. It should be noted that this trend was not an accidental one. It has resulted, at least in part, from the dialogues being carried out by Phoneticians (voice scientists), Laryngologists and Voice Pedagogists.

Beverley Johnson: I have found that most singers fear the terminology of the scientists; imagery seems to work better. Which is better, an empirical or a scientific approach? Perhaps a little of each is the answer. From the Symposia we have learned to blend the two and to use that which works best for the individual.

[…] I have been fascinated to learn that some of the doctors, researchers, and the scientists have actually been studying singing. One of my strongest feelings has always been that one cannot understand something until one has experienced it; and that is, I believe, especially so with singing.

[…] The larynx is one of the most complex organs in the body, and its functions are still imperfectly understood, despite much physiological and acoustical research. The use of the breath is also debated endlessly.

[…] Another major problem for the singer concerns the use of the so-called resonating cavities. There is much disagreement, some almost violent, about where the sound is shaped. In the last few years the majority of voice teachers have accepted the findings of the scientific investigators but have differed over the practical application of this knowledge. The fact that the scientific findings are admittedly incomplete has added to the confusion.

[…] To me, one of the most outstanding errors, in most systems of teaching, is that the student is plunged immediately into an attempt to control physiological and acoustical phenomena, without any accurate understanding of the subject. Here is one of the most important things the Symposia have done for us – giving us accurate measurements and understanding of these phenomena.

The 20th Anniversary Symposium at the Warwick Hotel in Philadelphia had three additional symposia added on over four days: 'State-of-the-Art Conference: Spasmodic Dysphonia', 'Neurolaryngology Symposium', and 'Objective Voice Measurements and Standards.'

The course objectives for all four symposia were:
- to provide information regarding recent technological, scientific and clinical advances in the study of the human voice;
- to provide information regarding diagnosis and treatment of voice disorders, and implica-

tions of vocal fold surgery;
- to increase understanding of various therapies and teaching techniques, as well as examination/evaluation of the voice, through workshops by recognized leaders in laryngology, speech pathology, speaking and singing;
- to foster dialogue and cooperation among otolaryngologists, speech pathologists, voice scientists, voice researchers, singing teachers, voice trainers, performers, and others who are concerned with care of the professional voice;
- to provide the latest information on diagnosis and treatment of spasmodic dysphonia (laryngeal dystonia);
- to provide interdisciplinary information about clinical and research aspects of neurolaryngology
- to increase understanding of the relationship of normal and abnormal voice production to acoustic, aerodynamic, muscular, respiratory, anatomic and videostroboscopic measures; and
- to foster appropriate selection, implementation, effectiveness and interpretation of laboratory measures by reviewing the advantages and limitations of current technology.

There was a special session on 'The Integration of Voice Science, Voice Pathology, Medicine, Public Speaking, Acting and Singing', and 'The Professional Speaker' was a special topic for a full day. 'Arts Medicine' was another special topic, and the G. Paul Moore lecture was 'Laboratory Advances for Voice Measurement' presented by Drs Gould, Korovin, and Pi-Tang Lin.

Almost twenty years later, Bonnie N. Raphael delivered the G. Paul Moore lecture at the 39th Symposium. She addressed advances, both accomplished and needed, such as how doctors better understand performers' needs, performers are going to doctors sooner, and how ENT doctors and voice scientists are publishing in the *NATS Journal* and VASTA's *Voice and Speech Review*. The following are excerpts from her lecture:

B Raphael, PhD: Each of us sees the world through a lens of perception that differs from culture to culture, from generation to generation, from gender to gender, from career to career, from individual to individual. Only when we can embrace our fundamental interconnectedness can our exchange of discoveries, ideas, theories and opinions reflect the true worth of Symposia such as ours.

[…] Now that scientists and doctors and therapists and coaches are taking interdisciplinary approaches to finding solutions, our perspectives are being enlarged and our horizons have grown far wider. It's a different paradigm; instead of seeking the one true path, we have begun to explore several doors into the same room in order to discover together many new and perhaps totally unforeseen possibilities. And sure enough, the whole is proving far greater than the sum of its parts.

[…] Some of us remain in danger of looking to 'prove' the value of a preferred methodology rather than honoring the rigor and validity of the scientific process.

[…] We continue to do our research on college undergraduates or clinical patients rather than with professional voice users, or even with MFA students in singing or in acting. I appreciate the difficulties inherent in attempting to do [research] in their environment instead of in labs, but if more researchers were willing to get out of their comfort zones, then their research might enter truly unexplored and more practical territory.

[…] Voice scientists might continue to move to more research on vocal athletes, and might undertake data collection under rehearsal and performance conditions, or at least conditions which more closely resemble those that actors and singers most often find themselves in.

[…] We still allow insurance companies to determine the length and extent of treatment according to criteria which are far from realistic for professional voice users.

[...] Much of what is taught to actors on a daily basis has not yet been verified by solid scientific data, collected under controlled conditions. We who teach need your help with the scientific study and evaluation of traditional and emerging systems of training, in order to move them from longstanding practice into the realm of proven validity and reliability.

[...] How are gender differences actually perceived by listeners? What are the most important ingredients of vocal transformation for transsexuals?

[...] The actor walks a dynamic tightrope between achieving enough of an emotional release to command an audience's attention and retaining enough control to be able to both structure a performance artistically and avoid cannibalizing him- or herself in the process. [...] Safe and efficient vocal performance that creates the illusion of distress without harming the voice requires the skillful combination of art and science. For this reason, it is important that medical advice, therapeutic advice and exercises, and performance coaching be not only useful, but realistic and custom-designed for each client.

[...] If I leave you with any final thought, it's that despite the discomfort of doing so (especially as we get older and more renowned), all of us can continue to grow by exploring beyond habit – by attending Symposium presentations and workshops outside of or only tangential to our particular fields of expertise and interest, by remaining open-minded regarding different doors into our rooms, by retaining a sense of curiosity and adventure rather than feeling we must defend our turf or reputation at all costs.

Back-Stories: *Bonnie Raphael, Mara Behlau, Harolyn Blackwell, Christine Sapienza*

Bonnie N. Raphael, PhD

Professor of Voice and of Dramatic Art, Head of the Professional Actor Training Program: University of North Carolina, Chapel Hill
Vocal Coach: PlayMakers Repertory Company
Vocal Coach: American Repertory Theatre, Harvard University

I grew up on Brooklyn, New York and I sounded like Edith Bunker. I got interested in theater; I was very young when I went to college, I graduated from High School at sixteen and from college at twenty. So I was very young, living at home and commuting by bus to Brooklyn College in New York. My parents were pretty conservative and they did not allow me to major in theater, even though that was an interest, so I majored in speech communication. My undergraduate degree is in speech education with a minor in theater. They let me go that far, but they did not want me associating with disreputable people.

Because of my undergraduate background I had a very good background in speech science and, when I chose my graduate school, I could have as easily gone into Speech Pathology as into theater. I decided on the theater side of things rather than Speech Pathology. But when I was looking around for a topic for my dissertation, one of my minors was in voice pathology, even on the PhD level. I was still taking courses in the Speech Pathology department and I wrote a dissertation on the relationship between characterization and functional voice problems in the actor. So I was sort of caught between two worlds: I wasn't a speech scientist, but I wasn't entirely a theater person either.

When I wrote my dissertation I had two dissertation advisors, which I do not recommend. One was in speech science, with a very rudimentary knowledge of theater, and the other was an acting teacher who knew virtually nothing about voice science. I was trying to write for both of them at the same time. It makes a better story than the actual experience.

Mara Behlau, PhD

ASHA Fellow
ASHA Certificate of Recognition for Outstanding Contribution in International Achievement
Permanent Professor: Departamento de Fonoaudiologia, Universidade Federal de São Paulo, Brazil

I'm first generation in Brazil. My mother was Italian, my father was German. When I ended my undergraduate program here I wanted to go to the US, but my mother didn't let me go because her city was bombed by Americans in the Second World War and she said, "No Americans." So I went to Italy. When I was there the Italians said, "Look, you should go and study in the US, because you have the profile of going and making things and there is this wonderful Italian-American professor, Oscar Tosi, that is at Michigan State University." So they sent me there. Since the Italians were sending me to the US, my mother accepted that. I went to do my Masters project on voice, because I wanted to work with voice. And then I saw a flyer for The Voice Foundation and I read it and said "Wow, it's a multidisciplinary approach! They have physicians, non-physicians, singers . . . I want to go to this place"!

My advisor was a physicist, so I was working hard stuff. And seeing something with singers and physicians was just wonderful, and so I asked him if I could go, and he said, "Ugh, those are a bunch of physicians that believe they understand voice. Voice is a physicist's domain. If you go, never talk to me on the meeting." Ok, I said, "Professor, I have to go because this is my first and only opportunity in the US." – I thought – "I'm not sure if I'm going to be able to come back to the US again, so I'm going to go."

So I went to my first Voice Foundation Symposium in 1983. It was in New York, at Juilliard, and Professor Wilbur Gould, the founder, was the chairperson and I was absolutely thrilled by it. Young Professor von Leden, young Professor Paul Moore were there giving classes. Friedrich Brodnitz, German-born, was there too. And I was absolutely enchanted by the possibility of having different perspectives on the same issue. And I said, "I have to go back. I have to go back." From 1983 to now, I just missed two. I do anything, but I never cancel The Voice Foundation.

First, when I decided to go to the university, I was interested in architecture – I thought it was very cool for a female. Then I was interested in psychology, but very abstract. And then I was very interested in law, but at that time in Brazil we were under a military dictatorship, and I thought, I'm first generation in the country, know nothing, this is not a good choice.

I wanted to do something in the health area, so I was considering medicine or speech-language pathology. I wanted to marry, to have four kids, and to have a part time job. I'm very bad on previewing the future, because just the opposite happened. I work from seven in the morning to ten in the evening, and two weekends per month, so it went all wrong. I have just one child, and more than one husband, so I did the opposite.

However, I am the most happy with my life and my unbearable agenda! And I love to be a therapist. I'm a clinician, I love the clinical job. Beyond voice, today I'm working a lot with communication for business. But this, everything is due to the voice area, and I went to voice because it was the one possibility of making me balance culture and science.

Harolyn Blackwell

Lyric Coloratura Soprano
Voice Faculty: Barnard College

My fourth grade teacher is responsible for helping me to become a singer. She was teaching a young boy soprano, who sang 'O Holy Night' during a concert with my 4th grade class. I was moved by the beauty of his voice. I discovered she taught piano and voice lessons. At first, I began with piano lessons. One day, she asked my mother whether she could also give me voice lessons along with my piano lessons. Once I began my voice lessons, I realized that singing was the best way I could express my emotions.

Ms Blackwell started on Broadway and then sang on many major opera stages around the world, including the Met, San Francisco, Chicago, Hamburg and Glyndebourne. She sang in many important concerts including one at the White House. She has an extensive discography including DVDs and television appearances.

Christine M. Sapienza, PhD

Dean of the College of Health Sciences, Program Director, and Professor, Communication Sciences and Disorders: Jacksonville University, Florida
Research Career Scientist: Malcom Randall VA Brain Rehabilitation Research Center, Gainesville

I was a student at the University of Buffalo and wasn't quite sure what I wanted to do. So, I took an undergraduate class, just to surf this area called speech and language pathology amongst other courses I was taking. The course was called Anatomy and Physiology of Speech and Hearing Mechanisms and Dr Elaine Stathopoulos was teaching the course. At the time, it was probably mid-career for her, she was up and coming, doing some interesting work in child respiratory function, and I just thought she was a really cool instructor. We met, and as a young student she took me under her wing. I think because she attended to what my intellectual needs were, we ended up striking up a really phenomenal mentor/mentee relationship.

Our relationship is what got me going in the area of respiratory kinematics, understanding child and adult differences, and learning about motor control theory. She had an NIH grant and I started working for her on the grant goals. She took me to conferences, introduced me to people that most didn't have the opportunity to meet, like researchers at Haskins labs. I got to do my first podium presentation at The Voice Foundation when I was a Masters level student. So, I stayed at UB the whole time – undergraduate, Masters, and PhD – mostly because I couldn't afford to go anywhere else. That was back in the day when they were funding graduate students to come to school, and Elaine helped get me into the Masters program, helped me get a fully funded line and I worked in her lab all the way until I finished my PhD.

She was the quintessential mentor. When I think back to that, I really don't know what I would've become without her. I was from a small town on the outside of Buffalo and I wasn't college-bred in any way. I didn't have parents that were encouraging me to be everything I could be. She really nurtured me by letting me know that I was an intelligent young woman and that there was opportunity if I worked hard. I try to convey that back to my students.

When I went to The Voice Foundation, Elaine introduced me to people like Ray Colton, Janina Casper, Bob Sataloff, Christy Ludlow, Tom Murray, Tom Hixon, Jenny Hoit, everybody who was hanging out in voice at that point, and they were all so kind to me. They just became kind of a support team. Then I graduated from Buffalo and went to the University of Florida, walked in, and there was Dr G. Paul Moore.

G. Paul Moore had been at Florida about twenty years, was the former chair of UF, and he still had his high-speed film lab. I moved into a little lab next to his. He was about eighty years old at the time and retired, but he was a Professor Emeritus and he still had very big lab space. Paul became my post-doctoral mentor, so here I was working almost another five years with him learning more about voice, about physiology, and doing voice clinic at Florida with Dr Mike Crary and Paul. Our work was like a snowball, we kept on working and building our team. When Paul gave up his lab space, I took over. I was extremely fortunate to ride on the shoulders of Dr Moore and other very famous people that took me under their wings. I learned from them.

At UF I also met Dr Paul Davenport, who is a respiratory physiologist and Dr Daniel Martin, a physical therapist, and somewhere in the late 1990s at UF, we got turned on to the development of a device for respiratory muscle strength training. That became a mainstay for us in terms of almost sixteen years of work. We put together this device for training expiratory muscles in people who had speech problems, problems with cough and, down the road, problems with swallow.

Somewhere in the early 2000's, I don't remember the exact year, two heavy hitters, Dr Michael Okun, a neurologist, and Dr Kelly Foote, a neurosurgeon, came to the University of Florida. They started a center for movement disorders which became a National Parkinson's Foundation Center and they incorporated speech pathology into their program planning. So they had physicians, nurses, and rehab, and we spent a lot of time studying Parkinson's, with funding through NIH, MJFox [The Michael J. Fox Foundation for Parkinson's Research], and Veterans Affairs. I just kept tripping over opportunity. I was at the University of Florida at a good time because they were on a big up-slope and lots of people were coming in, while at the same time I was given the opportunity to work with the historic and famous voice faculty like G. Paul Moore. University of Florida was an incredible twenty years of my career.

After serving as chair of the speech language pathology and audiology program for about eight years, I received a call from Jacksonville University. Jacksonville University (JU) is a private, high performing university sitting on the St. John's river. They asked me to come and start a new speech language pathology program. It has been an incredibly progressive time there and the individuals I work with in leadership are truly incredible.

We work with a lot of women in our field, and women today are a lot more confident than they were even ten years ago, but I think they all need to know that they are quite capable and that this is a field where they can make a high impact. And it doesn't mean you have to sacrifice your family values and your other personal choices. I try to help them figure out how to do that. The newer generation is called out less about it than they were in the past, but when I think about the doc students I mentored ten or fifteen years ago, some of them struggled with those choices.

You know, I don't even know sometimes how some of this stuff has happened. I'm a very positive person and I guess I have a mind that sees opportunity. I just don't look a gift horse in the mouth. If somebody is offering to mentor me, or offering for me to join a program, or offering me an opportunity to participate in a project or an event, I try to see where that may lead. I think I work really hard, and don't squander my time. I try to be very organized and if you're involved in ten opportunities and five of them end up being successful you look pretty good right? There's a lot of failure in there too. I've had grants that have been triaged and unfunded, and manuscripts that have been rejected, and sometimes students that go through problems, and my own family issues. It's not a perfect life in any way, but you keep the positive outlook. I'm a real believer in the mind helping you open up your own situations.

15

Breath – There Be Dragons

> The concept of defining variability within the bounds of acceptability is one of the important future aspects.
>
> R.C. Scherer, PhD

R.J. Baken, PhD: An important enduring mystery that cries out for resolution is the rules, if you will, of ventilatory control. There are all manner of beliefs and dogmas about breathing and speech or singing, but much of what I hear about the subject is, at best, assumption or speculation, and too much of it ignores – and in many cases violates – basic principles of physiology or even elementary physics. There also seems to be frequent confusion of cause and effect. The topic is the proverbial can of worms: we utterly lack, as far as I can see, a coherent theory of breath control for sound production.

Interestingly enough, in the early 1970s our lab at Columbia was heavily involved in studies of chest-wall control and we published a series of research articles. But we moved away from that area for a number of reasons, the most important of which is that we couldn't see light at the end of the theoretical tunnel. That is, as I said, we could see no emerging underlying theory coming from our research or that of the several others working in the area. For a scientist, not to have an underlying unifying theory is the baccia di morte. We got into some major disputes with Tom Hixon, some of them in print. The problem that I ultimately saw was that, even people like Hixon, who were very fine scientists and had been exploring the area for a long time, continued to find that, in many important ways, perfectly normal speakers and singers were largely idiosyncratic in their management of the air supply, often doing things that seemed inexplicably inefficient and counterintuitive. Which is what I mean by a can of worms. There seems to be no logical explanation for why person A does one thing, and person B something quite different under the same circumstances. Clearly the situation needs a lot of clarification.

B. Raphael, PhD: Tom Hixon reported on kinematic breathing research he'd done with actors from the Royal Shakespeare Company. He found out two fabulous conclusions: one was that voice teachers tend to teach others to breathe the way they do, but that the way people breathe is more directly related to their individual body type than to the absolute superiority of any one particular way of breathing for actors. Different body types breathe differently. Tall and skinny, you breathe in a different way than if you're short and stocky. And your tendency is to teach actors to breathe the way you do rather than the way they are physiologically built to breathe. I love that. I thought that was very useful.

The other thing was after actors from the Royal Shakespeare Company described in writing how they breathed, he wired them up with some kind of electrodes and he had them do a demanding Shakespearean monologue on stage. And he found that these very good actors from the Royal Shakespeare Company did not in fact breathe the way they said they breathed. And I found that extremely useful too.

That had me switch from teaching actors how to breathe to teaching them to breathe. Instead of prescribing any particular way to breathe, my attention shifted to making sure every new thought requires a new breath. So you're not breathing for physiological reasons, you're breathing for dramatic reasons. You're making the dramatic transitions during the intake of your next breath. And that was also very, very useful to my teaching.

K. Ardo: At the Symposia I was made very, very welcome. It was like a homecoming, a vocal homecoming every year. My training in Berlin with Dr Wolfgang Shütte was excellent, but being amongst all these medical people, I realized I should know a little bit more than just what I know of my own muscle memory. There was always a great discussion among different teachers about breathing and breathing techniques. I was pretty sure that my breathing was the correct way of breathing. I had to have core breathing because of my post-polio. I had to have the grounding, the feeling of equilibrium on a slanted stage when I couldn't feel my left leg on that slanted stage. So I had to work from that grounding of core. And you know I'd hear all these things about Miller and his open ribcage and holding the musculature and producing sound, and it was all in my head, going round and round. Then Dr Hixon presented at one of the Symposia about the results of his research of low abdominal breathing, low pelvic breathing, and core and I said, "Aha, yes! It is true, I'm doing it correctly!"

B. Raphael, PhD: I was participating in an experiment on voice fatigue with Ron Scherer at the Recording and Research Center in Denver. The second time we did this, I felt the task was too easy for a trained voice, so we had basically the same protocol except I had to do all the speaking on the same pitch. I was reading aloud from some voice dictionary or book, and everything I said was exactly on the same note, sustaining the same pitch and the same loudness for as long as I could. What we found out is, first my voice got better. Because they didn't let me warm up and I started cold. So the first 15 minutes and the second 15 minutes, my measurements actually improved. And then after that, I started fatiguing a little bit. And I can't remember how long the second time lasted, but the feeling I had in the sound proof booth is that I was running out of air. I just felt like I didn't have enough air to breathe. And afterwards, what we figured out was that my breathing muscles were tiring. I was supporting the voice, so I wasn't fatiguing my throat as much as I was fatiguing my breathing muscles.

We reported on stuff like that. I think they compared me with a lay person and with somebody who obviously had a clinical problem like Parkinson's. Then they lined up the three groups of data and this was an attempt to explore establishing norms for performers, as opposed to what passed for norms. It's like elite athletes who have a much lower pulse than normal people, things like that, much lower blood pressure. They didn't have norms for professional voice users, just norms for regular people. And the Voice Foundation has been pretty instrumental in bringing to the forefront the fact that there are different norms for professional voice users.

C. Sapienza PhD: What really is a supported tone and a non-supported tone? You know, I don't even know if it matters. To be honest, it's kind of a funny response, but people ultimately respond based on the quality that they hear. And I think there's lots of different ways you can configure the mechanics of the body to create that 'supported tone' or that 'unsupported tone.'

I think the body does what it's supposed to do, naturally. It doesn't like to work any harder than it needs to. Even the great Dr Tom Hixon, when he was studying respiratory mechanics with elite opera performers, they would think that X, Y, and Z were happening but, physiologically, they really weren't deviating that far from what would've been expected from the mechanics of the chest wall. I think the body moves with the minimal amount of physiological work, at the same time perceptually tuning into what it is that's being produced and what the auditory quality is.

I don't know if you can specifically train somebody to manipulate X plus Y plus Z. If ultimately a supported tone is one that is produced with high quality, and I think there's manipulations that go on in the oropharynx, larynx, and the respiratory system to paint it that are portative, plus your variables are different from me because of body type or size, plus your expectations are for your quality reaction from the audience and vice versa, it's multivariate.

Perhaps the definition is that it is different in everyone? Exactly. I agree with that.

R. C. Scherer, PhD: *Do you think there is ever going to be common ground on what a supported tone is and what is the correct way to breathe?*

There are two areas of information that are lacking. One is being able to measure and understand the control systems of the body for, in this case, making sound. The other is that there's undoubtedly a range of combinations of neurophysiological use that results in sufficient, adequate, and excellent results for voice and speech production. So, the concept of defining variability within the bounds of acceptability is one of the important future aspects to get a strong handle on.

It all comes down to understanding how the body works to make sound. We have to continue to have good ideas for that, good methodologies for that, and supportive research for that. When that happens – that is, the more precise the information, the more correct the ideas – two basic things will happen. The vocabulary that we use to talk about these things will change to more of an operational jargon and, secondly, the application will be much more precise, accurate, useful, and efficient.

J. Sundberg, PhD: Yes, I think we could measure a fair amount of things that would keep us busy for a number of years. I would like to understand placement and support; what does it mean, and does it mean the same thing to people? And could you synthesize an unsupported and a supported sound? That would be nice, because if we could synthesize it, we could describe it, but before that, it is going to be difficult. So that would be a missing piece of information – support and placement.

And then, of course, there are a lot of things: What is healthy vocal technique, tone production? What is a threat to the voice, and how do the successful singers do it? Is it a question of robustness of the organ, or is it a question of technique? And it must be both, I think. You could probably ruin any voice with bad technique.

It would be nice to derive from acoustic data, physiological information. I'm working at that now. Just by analyzing the output sound to be able to say that glottal adduction is too much here, and you need more airflow, or you need to add a bit of nasal resonance, or something like that. That should be fine to have.

16

In the Trenches

> You have a lot of possibilities to continuously vary the tone quality. And that of course is an important set of possibilities that singers are required to use in a meaningful way and if it is not meaningful, it's just bad singing.
>
> J. Sundberg, PhD

I. Titze, PhD: I know high level scientists in laboratories that don't have singers or clinicians in the group. They often produce academic results that publish well, but don't have anything to do with what's going on 'in the trenches.' You need to experience singing, you need to act or deliver speeches, to understand what is critical in vocalization. The best questions come from personal experience and struggles with your own voice.

The following quotations are answers and questions around practical information presented at the Symposia that stood out in the memory and could be directly used on stage and in the studio.

C. Hoffmann, PhD: Dr David Brewer introduced the Fiberoptic Scope to the Symposia, and an off-shoot coming from this was an experiment where I was asked to be a 'guinea pig.' With the scope in place, where we could see the vocal folds on the television monitor, I was asked to mentally hear a pitch without actually singing it aloud. It was amazing to watch the vocal folds adjust to the mental, unsung pitch and remain slightly open until the action of the sung pitch/vowel drew them into vibration. Singers are now advised not to practice silently when there is a vocal illness or injury because the vocal folds will track the pitches soundlessly and one needs to rest them from unnecessary activity. This new information also supported a tradition from the Bel Canto of hearing the pitch/vowel before producing it aloud to create a more harmonious coordination of the parts involved when one begins to sing.

C. R. Stasney, MD: Gould and Sataloff both took care of famous news anchors and taught them how to sing. They both thought it was important that professional speakers have good breath support. By teaching them to sing, they learned breath support and were able to project better.

J. LoVetri: There was a presentation (Xeroradiography with Electro-Laryngography) in 1981, by Dr Frances MacCurtain, whom I believe was from London, from The Royal College of Speech and Language Therapists. Her presentation was on work done with someone who had voice strain – I think what we would call now muscle tension dysphonia. She had made x-rays of two different people before and after they had therapy. And in at least one example, there was a huge difference in the 'before' and 'after' x-rays. I saw that in the first one, the person's tongue was cramped up and squeezed, the jaw muscles were really tight, and their soft palate was pulled up. In the second one, the 'after' shot, everything was relaxed and loose, and there was more physical room, more open space in the person's throat. I bought the transcript and still use it to explain to students that when we talk about functional difference, this is functional difference. It's not an imaginary thing. "Look at these x-rays! Look at the base of the tongue. Look where the larynx is. Look at the hyoid bone. Look at the epiglottis. See the difference. This is how our work is supposed to change a person's throat!"

―――――――

B. Raphael, PhD: Ingo Titze, who has been a mainstay of The Voice Foundation forever, taught this voice warm-up you can do through a straw that not only strengthens your breathing muscles but you can work full voice into a straw and it doesn't make much sound. So you can warm-up in a hotel room, or in a restroom adjoining the place where you're going to perform. There was so much that I learned from The Voice Foundation symposia!

―――――――

M. Benninger, MD: Some of the work with Richard Miller, that was part of my research block, was filming singers singing, which really hadn't been done to any great degree, and trying to figure out what happened to the larynx and the pharynx when people would create certain sounds.

The other thing Richard was working on involved his perception of his very good students, those that were expected to have a long career, versus his perception of the non-elite voices. Did they do things differently? Did the larynx look any different? I think the surprising thing for us was that they didn't.

―――――――

K. Ardo: I would love to research how to get the understanding of producing more energy from your body into making a better phonated sound, a supported, phonated sound. I hear myself repeatedly saying that you need more 'energy' to support a certain tone. Now, to explain this to a student, or even to a famous performer, is very difficult to put into words what you want them to do – how to get that airflow to phonate with energy. How do you do that? How do you connect to the core? How do you connect to your feet? How does one produce energy?

I have grown into this monster of thera-bands®. I use the strongest thera-band® that you can get your hands on, and also show them how to do their breathing with weights – which is very important for voice users. I'm getting all of these results, especially in older people who lack the energy from the diaphragm to be able to phonate and make a clearer sound. Even with some aging singers that are still performing, but are now worried with all of the hormonal changes. They're in their early sixties, wondering how do they continue to have and keep their energy? And I'm working with them on this thera-band® thing and it seems to be working.

―――――――

B. Raphael, PhD: I have been very forthcoming about actors learning how to do the wrong things the right way. In the past the speech pathologists used to say, "Oh you must never cough, if you can sniff and swallow instead, don't cough." Well, what if you're playing Camille who's dying of consumption? You gotta cough. So I've been teaching actors how to scream, how to shout, how to choke, how to laugh hysterically, how to sob. New things in the theater that the pathologists used to tell them, "Oh don't do that, don't do that at all," and now if you won't, somebody else will.

I also serve as an advocate for the actors. Actors are such people pleasers. You know they would turn themselves inside out to please a director. So a director says, "Can you do that?" "Yeah, of course I can." And what it's doing in many cases is what I call cannibalizing themselves. They're doing what they're doing at their own expense, and they can't do it forever. So occasionally, I will go to a director who is re-rehearsing and re-rehearsing a scene that is very physical, and the actor is being dragged around the floor and fighting or fencing or God knows what, and the director wants him to work at full energy. I will just say to the director – never publicly, you know – I pull him aside and say, "Could you just have the actor mark this for like the next half hour and then when you do the run through let him go full out?" Because directors don't think that way. So I have become much more of an advocate for the actors to the director, to the producer, who says, "Ah, so and so doesn't need a day off!" Then he gets a problem right before the show starts and the director says, "Oh, it's just stage fright, take some Xanax."

I am retired now, so I am doing less. But I teach with my scientific knowledge as a background. I am much more knowledgeable about the side effects from prescription drugs. Who thinks of asking the doctor, "Is this going to have an effect on my voice?' Or telling actors when you go in for surgery, you gotta have a talk with the anesthesiologist and tell them to use a smaller tube, tell them to lubricate it really well for intubation, and tell them to get it out of there as fast as possible. The doctor's not thinking about that, he's thinking about your broken leg.

So I've become much more assertive about actors' rights. You know, actors aren't that assertive about their rights. You know, sometimes a director says, "Oh I need a lot of London fog. This has got to be really moody. I want the lights really low, and lots and lots of fog." And depending on the chemical composition of that fog, it might be really bad for the actors to breathe. They don't think about stuff like that, or many of them don't.

I remember when I was at the Denver Center, the character in the play is supposed to smoke, and he's lying on the couch with his legs up and he's blowing smoke rings. And the door opens and his friend says "Oh I can always tell when you're here", because he can see the smoke rings. And the actor, God bless him, went down to the costume shop and asked for bunny slippers. He had some pretty outrageous bunny slippers. And he put them on his feet and he'd lay on the couch and he put up his bunny slipper feet and he, the guy says, "Oh I can always tell when you're here" and it got one of the biggest laughs in the entire show, and it had nothing to do with smoking.

So helping actors find the alternatives to smoking at all. Or, if they absolutely have to smoke, how to fool around with the cigarette, and play around with the ashes, and do everything except inhale. And that has been a big change in my teaching as well.

Resonance is another topic with slippery answers. Attempting to understand traumatic brain injuries, the Navy has been experimenting with massive percussive pulses aimed at gelatin-filled skulls to see what vibrates where. Perhaps the resultant knowledge could lead eventually to studying much finer pulses coming from within, to start to see just what is the elite singer feeling when they hit the sweet zone and it feels like the top of their head will fly off from the vibration.

R.H. Colton, PhD: Singers talk a lot about the feelings of resonance they experience when they sing. I don't think that should be ignored. That's a feeling, though. The sound could be transmitted through the bone, and we have done some work on that, have looked at the phenomenon of what the person is producing and what they are feeling. That is an important area. You need to look at the resonators, which are very important for voice people.

What we look at in the physical, acoustic world

and what the patient is feeling, are two different things. They are feeling things that we can't always measure. You can't measure the pain a person feels. You can quantify it to a certain degree, but we will always be limited in what we can measure. What some singers are feeling is hard to understand. We need to figure out where they are feeling it, and what are they really feeling? The vibration is in their nose, or jaw or ear? Different singers have different feelings. I'm trying to improve my golf swing, and you wouldn't believe the different advice I get about that. And that's much easier than singing.

———

I. Titze, PhD: Resonance. It is part of every description of voice, and we have examined the resonance qualities in the vocal tract. Singers have self-perceptions of resonances, feeling them in their head, cheekbones, jaws, etc., but those feelings (from vibration of tissues) do not relate strongly to what other people hear in our voice. Autoperception makes little difference eight to ten feet away. Experienced singers and vocologists understand this. There is still confusion about autoperception among singing teachers in high schools and churches.

———

J. A. Haskell, CCC-SLP: With an unlimited grant, I would explore vocal self-perception. I did my doctorate on this, and gave a half-hour TVF Symposium presentation. How people perceive their voices, and how can it be measured. I might think I'm speaking at a certain loudness level, and you might perceive it as a very different level. The same thing with pitch – I might think I'm talking awfully high, but you might perceive it as not so high, but in a normal range. I do a lot of informal work on how people perceive their voices, particularly when people come in thinking their voice is too high. Very often the voice is not too high, and the pitch is in a normal range, but for whatever reason, maybe the resonance, the inflection, or whatever. I think that is an area that has to be explored. Maybe someone will take it to the next step from my original study.

———

And then there are belting, rock and other CCM styles. There continues to be debate and dissatisfaction about what exactly is belt production, and Broadway is not cooperating by changing what it is looking for on a regular basis. The belt needed for *Mame* is not the one needed in *Wicked*, although they both need a powerful belt. Belt styles (not surprisingly) fall into the same categories that musicals have fallen into: Classical, Disney, Pop, Rock, Gospel, etc. When asked about voce di sprega (or belting) during a NATS CHAT in November 2014, Dr Sataloff added his voice teacher hat to his physician's coat and the following is excellent advice for anyone wish to belt.

———

R. T. Sataloff, MD, DMA: There are lots of misconceptions about belting. The first thing someone needs to understand about belting, no matter what other technical approaches one wants to take, is that great belters are not shouters. Whether we are talking about the current high-belt trend in adults, or whether we are talking about these poor eight to eleven year-olds trying to sing Annie, if you listen to the ones who end up in our offices, they have a fairly constant volume with little change in vocal output, and are essentially shouting.

When we teach classical music, in addition to teaching technique, we often encourage people to listen to recordings of great artists. If you are teaching a tenor, you will want that person to listen at one time or another to Pavarotti, Gigli, Bjorling, Melchior, and to listen to a range of techniques and finesse, on different notes.

In the belting world, people need to pick up the Ethel Merman recordings. If you listen to and study a great belter, and I think people will agree that Merman was as great a belter as we've had. You will have trouble finding a single note that is the same from beginning to end. Her variation, note by note, whether it is volume, vibrato, pitch, or all of them, is infinite. So if people are going to belt at all, and especially if they are going to try and carry a belt mechanism higher than it should be, at the very least they should be doing it with very distinct variation in the voice on practically every note they sing.

Most singers can create that same kind of belt effect by inflection and by style, rather than by carrying the laryngeal position of chest voice into the highest notes, and the audience can't tell the difference. And it is much easier and much safer. That's what I recommend, whether people learn how to do that and get that style without it suddenly going from belt to sounding too legit, or not, they do it using a more legit technique stylized. If they do it loud all the time, then they are going to end up in your office or mine.

During this same online NATS CHAT, Dr Sataloff answered questions from voice teachers, giving them useful, practical advice. One of the recurring topics is hormone replacement therapies. Singers and teachers are justifiably concerned about the changes in voice quality and range, for men and women, with andropause and menopause.

Another major concern among elite women singers is what happens when a woman has a hysterectomy and is sent into early menopause? Gynecologists do not tend to take the voice into consideration, and it can be difficult to find a doctor who understands what surgery will do to the upper range and flexibility of the voice. The most recent research on these topics is regularly presented at The Voice Foundation Symposia.

L. Carroll, CCC-SLP: I think The Voice Foundation does a better job of disseminating critical information and advances on how to care for and manage the voice than many of the pure singing organizations do, because it is interdisciplinary. When you have a convention that is just of one discipline it is hard to think 'outside of the box' and how that relates to 'inside the box.' TVF has always been about being all-inclusive and now it's not just performance voice, but all manner of voice use.

There is remarkable, practical, usable-in-the-studio and onstage, information presented at each TVF Symposium, and the question is: how to get the information out where voice professionals, and their teachers and coaches can find it? Dr Sataloff and Dr Ingo Titze write regularly for the National Association of Teachers of Singing's *NATS Journal*, with articles by Dr Sataloff appearing in nearly every issue. TVF and TVF scientists helped NATS with its August 2014 Vocapedia launch, and is adding two articles from each issue of the *Journal of Voice* to the Vocapedia database.

Here are a few responses to the question, "How do we get the word out?"

H. Blackwell: I would say, to get the word out to voice teachers, coordinate with NATS. The Classical Singer conference should also have a TVF presence. Perhaps one of the basic medical presentations could be offered? And have you thought about a presence at AARP conferences for help with and information about changes due to aging in the voice?

The biggest thing that I have discovered is the care of the voice when students are sick. Often, I have to explain to them about medications and foods that might cause problems for their voices. Many of them aren't aware how delicate the voice is and what it takes to maintain a healthy singing and speaking voice.

M. Hawkshaw, CORLN: I would like more awareness of just what The Voice Foundation is, why it exists, and who benefits from it. I think we need to reach out to television personalities, broadcasters, and the like. Some people are born with a fantastic voice and just know how to use it, but I would like to see more education of the lay population.

We also have to consider all these voice

competitions like *American Idol*, *The Voice*, this and that, *America's Got Talent*.' Are they overdoing it? Are they good for young voices?

J. LoVetri: I would like TVF to be a little bit less conservative in what it says about itself. The Voice Foundation has broken so much ground. Having the CCM panel in 2006 was breaking huge amounts of ground! No one had done that before. But who knows today that we did that? If a marketing company was hired to market The Voice Foundation and the Symposium, they would want to emphasize the truth about all the breakthroughs, all of the original ideas that have gone on to fruition, that started at the Symposium. I think that would make The Voice Foundation stand out. It would help make it more imperative for the young doctors, researchers and singing teachers to have to show up.

W. Riley: There is a lot happening now because of the internet. There is a greater sense of knowledge and comfort with technology. People who are not really scientifically trained in universities are beginning to look at this information. That is a two-edged sword. First of all, getting access to the information and being able to quote chapter and verse on research, doesn't mean that you really understand it. A lot of people are beginning to quote research, sometimes out of context, and they don't really apply it correctly.

So, The Voice Foundation plays a very important role in educating people about what all of these things really do mean. You can't just say certain things and expect them to be true. You have to understand them. TVF still is the place where researchers remind people that if you have a process that is automated, and you push the button and get a result, you really have to be able to calculate those numbers by hand, too. TVF teaches the younger generation to do those hand calculations.

Ron Baken was the first to tell Linda Carroll, "You can't trust a machine to do what a scientist can do" and the world of speech pathology and even medicine, wants to trust the machine. We need to train people to not always trust the machine, and know how to calculate the number itself, from scratch – especially if the number doesn't make sense to you. The Voice Foundation exists as an educational entity primarily to preserve the integrity of the voice and voice research.

M. Behlau, PhD: I think that The Voice Foundation should be having online sessions all over the world. Not the whole Symposium, but some sessions could be broadcast online via computer, as a pay-online congress. Many people cannot go to the Symposia, it's too expensive for them, but I'm sure if they were offered, they would buy. We could have sessions, with subtitles in other languages, have classes and presentations on the internet, on YouTube.

The Voice Foundation could have a channel on the voice with those kind of files that you cannot copy, etc., that you can see by payment. A small payment that The Voice Foundation can benefit from. I think that The Voice Foundation should go online for some sessions and should produce more interactive content, like quizzes, cases on the internet, tests on what a speech-language pathologist should know about vocal pedagogy, what a teacher of singers should know about vocal habilitation, what everybody has to know about surgery, and so on.

Maria Russo: For me, the key to the future of The Voice Foundation and the challenge for the Executive Director, is to simultaneously maintain the unique atmosphere of warmth and excited exploration and to survive and grow in today's world. To stay relevant and remain the leader in interdisciplinary cooperation and research, TVF will need the same kind of passionate dedication and grand personalities that initiated this commixture. We need to rouse related disciplines to join the fun. Loyal membership allows us to exist, but continued existence is not enough. It's a tall order to ask people to invest even more when everyone is busy beyond capacity.

'If You're Not Constantly Moving Ahead, You're Falling Behind.'

TVF started as a relatively small group effort with funding generated by connections to large corporations, and the gala atmosphere of the time in NYC. For many reasons, those paths are not as lucrative as they were. It has been essential to move from a small, club-like structure to an organization which is not simply professional and self-sustaining, but growing, without losing the sense of being on a shared adventure. The Philadelphia team did much of that in the years after the organization moved and I think we've even done more in the past few years. We added social media and a more sophisticated website, an email service, and some videos to the already daunting duties of managing *Journal of Voice*, Membership, Boards, Committees, Awards, Symposium, Gala, World Voice Day events, publicity, advertising and grant writing. Adding a membership area to the website and adding chats and more videos are on the agenda. However, quite simply, more projects require more staff. So, how do we implement growth on the reduced funding available to non-profits today? That is the question for us in the office, the Board of Directors, and for all members.

In the Strauss opera *Capriccio*, the poet and the composer, Olivier and Flamand, debate the relative powers of words and music. In the endeavors of TVF the question is moot. It's the ability of the voice, spoken or sung, to communicate, stir our emotions, intoxicate and inspire, and even heal us that moves TVF members to continue the quest to understand how it works and to be able to help and heal the voice in return.

Back-Stories: *Michael Benninger, Jeannette LoVetri, Peak Woo*

Michael S. Benninger, MD, FACS

Otolaryngologist
Cleveland Clinic
Henry Ford Hospital
Chair: Head and Neck Institute, Cleveland Clinic
Professor of Surgery: Cleveland Clinic Lerner College of Medicine, Case Western Reserve University
President: International Association of Phonosurgery

Becoming a doctor was kind of strange. I was a football coach, actually, and a biology major in college. And after two years coaching college football, I decided that that probably wasn't for me. My original plans were to go into marine biology because I was at Harvard and they had Woods Hole and the Marine Biology Institute, but there were no jobs there. My roommate had gone to medical school and he said you may want to consider it, so I spent a little time at Mass General Hospital and then said: OK, this works for me.

In terms of getting into voice and laryngology, when I was a third-year resident I had to do a research block and Howard Levine, who was one of our Attendings, basically said "Hey I've got a research idea for you. There's this teacher of music out at Oberlin Conservatory of Music that would like to start doing some research with us and I don't have time to do it. How would you like to be the point person on that?" And that person was Richard Miller, who was a very famous pedagog and music teacher. He and I spent the next year or so, on and off, doing all kinds of early research in voice which actually prompted my first presentations at The Voice Foundation in around 1986, when I first presented the work that we had done together.

By the time I finished my residency, there were very few people in the mid to late 1980s that were focusing on non-cancer voice, or larynx. I went to Detroit, with its dynamic music scene. There were still a lot of the old Motown people there, the new 1970s and 1980s rockers, like Bob Seger and Mitch Rider, and all these up and coming people like Madonna, Kidd Rock and Eminem. In addition, the Michigan Opera Theater, the big opera company there, had just purchased one of the old downtown movie theaters and were renovating it into a beautiful opera house. So that all kind of just came together and propelled my interest in voice and laryngology.

I was introduced to laryngology through Richard Miller, Howard Levine, and Harvey Tucker, who was a laryngologist and my Chairman, so I had that early exposure to laryngology. But really, it was going into Michigan and being able to do it on my own. I was there with a couple of very famous speech pathologists, just by chance, one of whom is Barb Jacobson. Barb Jacobson and I developed something called the Voice Handicap Index, a quality of life instrument that is used to assess the impact of voice on overall quality of life. She and Alex Johnson were there with me, and after three or four years we decided to write a book on performance voice, *Vocal Arts Medicine, The Care and Prevention of Performing Voice Disorders*. I have now published two additional books related to performing voices and another to be out soon.

Jeannette L. LoVetri

Founder and Director: The Voice Workshop
Creator: Somatic Voicework
Secretary: The American Academy of Teachers of Singing

When I was twenty-two years old, living in Connecticut, I agreed to be vocal director for a production of *Finian's Rainbow* I worked with the whole company, with the chorus and the individual singers, teaching them the music in the show. Some of them asked me for private lessons, so I thought: "OK, I have already been studying for seven years. I can try taking them on as private students." You can be very confident when you are young and don't know any better!

The following summer, I vocal-directed another musical, *Once Upon a Mattress*, and had the same experience. The students in the show became my next private students. Then, other people who knew I was teaching occasionally sent me more people and, before I knew it, I had a small group of students coming to study at my house.

I moved to New York in 1975, my studio grew, and in 1980 I got my first Broadway students. One of them was playing the role of Peggy Sawyer, a lead in the production of 42nd Street that was revived that year. She sent me other Broadway people, and that's how I got involved in musical theater in New York.

Around that same time, I started teaching at a small private college in East Orange, New Jersey. It was a mix of classical and musical theater students. That's how I became a full time singing teacher. I haven't performed professionally since 1979, although I occasionally sing in public, both classically and in CCM styles. My original training was classical, and I attended the Manhattan School of Music as a classical voice major but I didn't like it. I was unhappy there, so I quit. All of the rest of my training was done on my own in private lessons and classes in adult education. I did different kinds of things in different places, working with a variety of teachers and coaches.

A lot of my early performing experience was in music theater. When I came to New York City, I did some off-Broadway shows which were pop/rock/gospel oriented. I sang for about five years with that same core group of people in different venues here in New York – at Lincoln Center and Rockefeller Center, and St. Peter's Church. I did some recitals, oratorio solos and some original classical pieces that were written for me at that same time.

I went to my first Voice Foundation Symposium in 1978 at Juilliard and met several teachers there who were members of the New York Singing Teachers' Association, who asked me if I'd join, so I became a member. Then in 1980 I joined NATS, met other colleagues and went to conferences and became more seriously committed to being a really competent teacher and going to The Voice Foundation Symposia every year.

In 1988, I was invited by Dr Sataloff to teach a workshop on music theater singing training. After that workshop, Johan Sundberg commented, "I've never seen anybody go from belting to classical sounds to 'mixing.' I think this is fascinating. If you ever are in Sweden I would love for you to come to the lab and let me see what it is you're doing."

I thought, "Well, this sounds like an opportunity that would only come once in a lifetime!" By then, of course, I knew who Johan was. I had read his 1977 article in *Scientific American* years before, and I actually had private tutoring to understand what he wrote in this article because I found it quite difficult, but knew it was important to comprehend.

That fall, I asked a student of mine in Copenhagen to arrange a workshop for me, and then arranged with Johan to come to Malmo, Sweden, afterwards for five days. Dr Patricia Gramming and Dr Sundberg did research on my vocal production. They spent all day, every day for five days, looking into my throat and having me sing.

I was able to stay in Dr Sundberg's home with his family, and have the great advantage of personal tutoring with this amazing man for five days. I asked him all kinds of questions about what was in his book, and what it meant, and what I was seeing in my throat, and what he was looking for, and why did that matter? And I learned an amazing amount in those five days.

At that time, the fiberoptic scope was large and cumbersome and the camera was enormous. It wasn't fun having that go in and out of my right and left nostril for five hours at a time, especially without anesthesia because I was afraid it might skew what I was doing.

Yet it was an exceptional experience having them show me the formant changes and how different the formant configurations were from mixed (register) to belting. This is why I think I get disturbed about people who are teaching belting who have no clue what they are doing. They make up, based on their subjective impressions, what they think is happening, without really knowing. The information I received then and subsequently, through a lot more study, clarified that the vocal production is not the same as classical singing. It produces different resonance characteristics because it's an entirely different vocal production!

In addition, Dr Gramming, an ENT, was able to inform me about all the structures that I was seeing in the throat and what they did and where they were. So I came back in 1987/8 with this 'graduate school' education in my head from being with them. I also spent a number of days, over a period of a few years, in Dr Sataloff's office watching him treat patients and watching his faculty work with people. That was also incredibly informative for me.

In 1999, I did a vibrato study with Ingo Titze and had access to him for four days. I asked him eight million questions about this and that, and then watched his research with the other people in that study. They actually stuck electrodes in my throat, in the thyroarytenoid and the cricothyroid muscles. I made sound while they ran electricity through my vocal folds. If you really want to know what's going on in your throat you can have that experience!

That was also an enormous gift and, yes, it was frightening to have someone else vibrating your vocal folds with electricity but it was also something I chose to do and I had no negative side effects when it was over.

Peak Woo, MD, FACS

Otolaryngologist
Clinical Professor of Otolaryngology: Icahn School of Medicine at Mount Sinai
Director: Grabscheid Voice Center, Mount Sinai 1996–2008

The physician for my residency in Boston, was Dr Stewart Strong. He was a throat specialist, and back in the 1970–80s, he developed a laser for surgery of the vocal folds. As a resident working with Dr Strong, we were seeing singers and other voice professionals who would fly in from New York and other cities to see him. At that time, there were very few people doing surgery of the throat. So as a resident, I often had the opportunity to work them up – fairly well known people, opera singers and rock and roll singers, and it just seemed really neat that here was a physician who was also the chair, who was uniquely gifted in this new technology to treat these singers who were otherwise in distress. That whole idea that you could help them, and get almost instantaneous voice improvement, was very attractive. So that was the impetus to think that, wow, this is a pretty cool new field.

Mid 1970s and late 1970s, another professor, Charles Vaughan, would take one of his residents (i.e. me) down to The Voice Foundation Symposium at Juilliard. A lot of artists, even music critics would come. They would have a much less scientific discussion about what was voice; How do you treat voice problems, singer's problems? It was more of an open forum discussion back then. It was interesting, because this was an area that very few people knew anything about. So that was also an interest, thinking "You could make a difference." So I think those were the two things that got me interested.

17

To-Do List

If you had the perfect grant, what would you study? What needs further clarification or research?

R.C. Scherer, PhD: What still needs to be clarified? The short answer is everything. We tend to be most interested in the eventual application to improving people's lives or satisfying their desire for certain skills. There's a short term and a long term aspect to this. The short term is related, I think, to communicating more effectively the existing information that is fairly accurate, so that practitioners don't make the mistake of using outmoded concepts and inappropriate methodologies.

The long term is to do the more difficult research to clarify how the body works to make sound. That has many dimensions from the neurological, physiological, psychological, etc., Also, the different disciplines need to be more clear about what each other does, what their needs are, how one can help them with those needs at the present time, and clarify, across the disciplines, the ideas that are most accurate.

Meetings like The Voice Foundation Symposia and the other kinds of more focused meetings are critically important for sharing and mutual learning. We really enjoy working with colleagues and students from other professions to help share information about voice science and vocal health, and do what we can to help each other solve immediate problems. And long term, we need to enhance the theories, the concepts, and the research methods that better solve the problems more permanently.

P. Woo, MD: Neural control of the vocal tract as well as intrinsic muscles of the larynx. The neural control of vocal fold movement is still not very well understood. We still don't know a lot about the neural physiology of those small muscles in the vocal cords. That's an area of basic science that has not gotten a lot of study in the last ten to fifteen years. There is a lot of interest now in vocal cord microstructure, a lot of interest in the lamina propria, a lot of interest in the different chemistry of the cells and layers, but we are still in the infancy in terms of understanding the neural control of vocal cord function. That is a pretty big area, that is a bit difficult to study easily because you often use animal models, and there is a large movement away from animal studies.

R. T. Sataloff, MD, DMA: We need to develop:
- much more accurate and much more sensitive acoustical measures;

- we also need some advances in aerodynamic measures;
- we could do better in standardizing perceptual evaluation; and
- we're not doing well at all in clinical measurements of size and anatomy of the vocal fold edge. That's another place that needs development, but
- the biggest and most challenging is acoustic signal assessment.

What do you think needs to be researched? One of our most vexing problems is vocal fold scar, which is essentially an issue of healing. Healing science needs to be advanced so that we understand how to prevent the development of unfavorable scar; how to predict its development, probably on the basis of genetic analysis; and how to repair unfavorable scar, ideally by genetic regeneration of the superficial lamina propria. That probably is our biggest clinical challenge.

M. Behlau, PhD: There are two levels of need. We still need basic stuff, such as normal data on voice and larynx all over the world, and on the opposite of this continuum, we need multi-centric studies on treatments. So, we need controlled clinical trials with several types of treatments, several types of dysphonias, multi-centric all over the world. And the opposite, we still need work on the fundamentals: What is a normal voice? What is a normal larynx? What is asymmetry, symmetry? Up to what point a rough voice, a breathy voice can be considered normal or deviated? We need evidence: randomized, controlled, clinical trials.

We need to clarify the limits between normal variations, stylistic variations, and deviation. What are the limits between normal variability of vocal quality and a degree of vocal deviation? What is the vocal deviation due to a style or due to a preference? Brazilians prefer low, breathy voices. If I go to the US, like in central Texas, they prefer high-pitched female voices. High-pitched female voices in Brazil, they don't survive. We hate women that 'meow' here; we tend to reject high pitched voices. Brazilians speak low pitch because we love that. I think cultural preference, vocal styles, and deviations that are risky to the vocal health are still something that needs to be clarified. And limits of vocal rehabilitation and limits of surgery too, because sometimes we don't know the limits on that, and it's very hard. I would adore working on different programmatic approaches to voice rehabilitation to produce data.

And I also would like to understand brain changes before and after rehabilitation; neural changes, central neural changes before and after rehabilitation on the voice; MRIs to see the brain effects with vocal rehabilitation. The voice is such a heavy identity, such a strong identity. When you change a voice due to vocal rehabilitation or after a disease, after a cancer, after a neurological impairment such as vocal fold paralysis – what happens in your brain? What happens in your vocal identity? So I would adore seeing brain changes with diseases and after treatment.

We have wonderful MRI research before and after Lee Silverman Voice Treatment (a treatment for patients with Parkinson's disease) that has shown that there are differences in brain configuration and concentration after treatment. But there are just a few studies.

C. Sapienza, PhD: I think we need to keep working on defining treatment effectiveness. As a field, I don't think we've done a tremendous job at looking at efficacy and effectiveness of the best of our voice and swallow treatments. A part of it is that our funding agency is so small we just don't get enough money to have large RCT's going on and multi-site trials. If we were doling out pharmacologics, people would expect it, but we dole out these behavioral treatments and people don't feel threatened if they don't work out right. Any side-effects or potential harmful effects of our treatments aren't grave. So, I don't know if we need clarification as much as it is betterment.

R. H. Colton, PhD: Some recent experiments didn't give us what we were expecting. Sometimes you get a negative result or no result, and editors tend to not want to publish that. I think it can be instructive and informative to find out what didn't happen, but journals won't publish these papers. I don't see the reason why people should rediscover the sun.

R. C. Scherer, PhD: We need so much more relative to the relationship of muscle function and structural movement, and the resulting motions, pressure, flows, and acoustics. So the neurophysiological aspect is a field that really needs a great deal of work. Even basic EMG studies need to be done much more.

Another area of study is still the respiratory management of air pressures and airflows relative to sound production. We can't devise the most efficient ways of training people and rehabilitating people and finding out what optimal coordinative activity is without this. It is important to understand how to define the range of efficient body function when producing healthy but on target voice and speech.

C. Hoffmann, PhD: When meeting students during a first-time consultation, I have observed that many have a lack of anatomical knowledge. This is a surprise, that the information on the location of the diaphragm, lungs, etc., is not more thoroughly understood by students today. There is an important difference between the perception of what is happening when we breathe and the physical reality that causes the movement of the parts involved – where the diaphragm is located and attached, its angle in the body, the lungs and their location, etc.

We need to know more about the right brain–left brain function in singing and speaking.

Has there been a discussion of the frenulum, and the vocal issues involved when this membrane is too short to allow the independent articulation of consonants by the tongue without engaging jaw tension? This problem seems often overlooked.

More detailed study of the Alexander Technique and its application, long and short term. How the relationship of the head, neck and body (lengthening and widening) can change the inner relationships of palate and jaw, alignment, breath, and neural connections to the spine, etc.

More study of the agonist/antagonist action as it relates to vocal registers and the management of the same.

M. Hawkshaw, CORLN: I would have to say voice education at an early age, like in grade school, high school and college. Everybody teaches how to get up in front of the class and give a speech, or give a lecture, but nobody teaches how to use your voice.

That's my biggest issue, that there are no required courses. That's what I would like to see. We teach them how to read, we teach them how to write, but we don't teach them how to speak. Often children learn to sing, play instruments but we don't teach them how to speak and use their voice or 'breathe' during such endeavors. If you're going to be a professional voice user, athlete, or if you're working in industry where there's a lot of noise, you need to know how to use your voice effectively in all these different environments.

The number one population of patients we see with vocal fold pathology are teachers; i.e., classroom teachers and choral directors, to name a few. Classroom teachers to coaches, who are out on the field shouting to lacrosse players, or football players. Noone is taught how to yell correctly.

We've made great strides in the treatment of papilloma and vocal fold scar; there's still more research to be done there.

H. Blackwell: An area that needs to be further addressed is the menopausal and andropausal voice. Some of my colleagues have had early menopause, and needed help in how to adjust to this problem, because many are still performing and teaching.

This subject is just starting to be addressed, but it is a huge issue and singers need more information. Many singers get to this point in their careers and wonder: What is happening? What do we do? What exercises? What do we need to do health-wise?

As singers, whether female or male, menopause and andropause are a major stage in careers and in our lives, and NATS, Classical Singer, and The Voice Foundation have begun to address this issue. With the help of these institutions, I am hopeful that more will be done by asking the questions and finding the answers to empower singers at this stage in their careers and lives.

———————

B. Raphael, PhD: One of the things that I was pleading for was research in situ. It's much easier to do research in labs. It's like going to a speech pathologist, and the actor is describing his problems and the speech pathologist says, "Well, why don't you do it for me now the way you do it on stage." And the actor gives it his best shot, he really does, but it's nowhere close. So any experimentation or research that could be done with the actor during performance, or in rehearsal, I think would be much more difficult to design, but much more valuable to the practitioner.

Questions that I would love answered from the scientists are about how long is the ideal warm-up? Are there any vocal ways of teaching that are superior to others? Basic questions that are harder to address.

Please provide some people who know what they're talking about and can translate the graphs and the statistics into terms that we can understand. They're talking to each other rather than the entire assembled group. That has been one of my soap boxes.

———————

J. LoVetri: We have zero information on the effect of microphones and monitors on vocal output. Every professional CCM singer needs a really excellent microphone, a great monitor, and hopefully a decent sound system or sound engineer, because they affect the sound as you're making it. That's so important and we haven't looked at it at all yet.

If someone were to come to me and ask, "What are the normal range and acoustic parameters for a 35-year-old male gospel belter?", I would be able to answer based on my life experience as a teacher, but I can't say, "Go get this article, or go get this book, or go look this up" because there is no such data. We do not have baseline measures or normative data on any contemporary commercial music style for any age range of professional singers."

Research on college students and college faculty is of no use to us at this point. I would like to see us research people who have been singing successfully for twenty, or twenty-five, or thirty-five years. I want to know what Tony Bennett's (or one of his colleagues) throat looks like. I want to know what anybody who has been singing for twenty-five or thirty years and still sings well is doing. The longevity factor, in terms of the real world, matters. And that's true in all of the performing arts. Generally, you don't sing Norma when you're twenty-two years old. And you don't dance the Swan Queen when you're eighteen years old. You don't do King Lear when you are twenty-five. You don't do things at those ages that you can do at fifty! (And, vice versa.)

There are some music theater roles that are risky for young belters to sing because they are quite hard, vocally and physically. Even if you have a really excellent belter, her body and throat may not have the stamina to be able to sing something demanding eight times a week in a Broadway show. I say this due to my 40 plus years of life experience as a singing teacher, but not because of scientific research in this area. I understand that it may not be easy to do research in the field as I am requesting it, but that is where we have to go now.

A number of years ago I attended a presentation about choral research. Afterwards, I asked if all the research had been done on collegiate choirs. The answer was "Yes." What about a chorus like the Metropolitan Opera Chorus? Or Covent Garden?

Has anyone ever studied those choruses? Those choruses are the professional ones, and some of those members have been there for thirty years. Don't we want to know what they're doing with their throats?

A Voice Bank of Proven, Experienced Voices: I've spoken to several people about the possibility of a library of sound bites of professional singers in each style. If that were possible, then anybody doing acoustic research or perceptual studies, anywhere in the world, could go to this library and access consistent professionally viable sounds in any style. That would make consistent data more likely and a broader base of information could be collected from professionals rather than college students or faculty.

Here is an example: if five men and five women who were Broadway belters with ten years of professional experience, sang Happy Birthday in two consistent keys, at a certain decibel level, or at a certain distance from an iPhone, and all of those recordings were stored in that library, with the examples marked singers 1,2,3,4,5 … 10, with no names, everyone could access these samples for research purposes. Then record gospel singers, country western singers and singers of all styles in the same way, collecting these samples from people all over the world who are professional singers, performing for ten years at a high level (such as in an A or a B house or an equivalent venue), and add those samples to the library.

This would also be the criteria of what belting is, because the samples would be from long-standing high-level professionals. I think it would level the playing field and help end the argument about what belting (or any other vocal quality) is and is not, as the marketplace would have made the determination.

J. Rubin, MD: Redevelopment of the lamina propria. I think it's difficult but I think it's certainly within the realm of possibility. The problem is that we have materials that are very similar to the lamina propria, for example hyaluronic acid, but the body absorbs them. The problem with, or the beauty of, the amazing thing about the larynx, is it's extraordinary durability, that it can vibrate so many times with relatively little damage – and that we get so much diverse use of it. It's really an amazing structure. It's so small, the vocal folds are only about two centimeters I mean they're tiny!

Voice is still a young science. We really need to know more about how to recreate the larynx. The whole area of stem cells and how they fit in is fascinating. Particularly, how to recreate the lamina propria, what to do after it has been damaged or destroyed, how to deal with scar. How to recreate a damaged vocal fold – that's really the critical thing. Or if you have somebody who has a paralyzed vocal fold, how to get that vocal fold functioning again. Those are crucial issues. Steven Gray was a leader in these areas; His students and coworkers, who are many, still name him on their scientific papers. And of course, he was another protégé of Jim.

Oh, there's still a lot of work that needs to be done. The field of robotics, I think, is something we will be getting more involved with in the near future: for example creation of a vocal device that's understandable, that can be talked to externally and can respond. I'm sure that we're just at the beginnings of robotics, and the vocal aspect of robotics will become very important.

C. Sapienza, PhD: I would like to see more done with regard to what our treatment actually, mechanistically, imposes. We do a lot of pre-assessment and we do a lot of post-assessment but we don't get a lot of sense for what goes on during. It's challenging both from an expense standpoint and from a methodological standpoint, how to really study human behavior, and how to study the human brain and how it adapts within therapeutic strategies. We don't really see the full dimension of brain plasticity. We don't necessarily have easy tools to examine cerebral blood flow, and to be looking at the central nervous system and the peripheral nervous adaptations that go on when people are exposed to therapeutic interventions or strategies. That's cool. If you could be doing all of that in real time, and be able to look at the physical and emotional side of human response to therapy, that would be awesome.

With the 'perfect grant', I'd bring all the neuroimaging people together with all the people who do biomechanical modeling with all the people who do really good physiology, and then all the speech language pathologists and physicians that actually have to figure out how to treat the patients. Put them all together in one room and tell them to tell us what it is we're actually affecting when we impose a treatment.

Can you watch the brain and can you biomechanically model for me when I do a voice therapy, or a swallow therapy? What am I actually doing in the lower airway and in the pharynx? What's going on with the tongue? What's happening at the palatal level? You know if you could just see all that, if you could actually be watching all of the physiological and muscular and cortical adaptations as if you could see through the patient. If you could watch their body response, at the same time knowing if they're engaged or happy, or what their emotional response was. I think there's a lot to the placebo-effect: there's a lot to the mind, it would be cool to be watching what the emotional placebo was that was going on.

It's just a few people who are starting to do functional magnetic imaging to be able to look at that connectivity. It's tough stuff to design. It's expensive to do. You can only sample a certain window of time and you can only translate so much of it to the real environment. I think we'll get there, we're a lot farther than we were, but the connectivity and the adaptations that go on would be fun to study.

———

J. Sundberg, PhD: I would buy some contemporary equipment because equipment is important and facilitates recording, and then I would like to have an anechoic chamber so I could get the clean signal and not a lot of room reflections polluting the signal recorded and analyzed. And then I would like a secretary for the first time in my life. That would be wonderful, to help me keep track of what I'm doing. And then I would like to hire a doctoral student or two, and guide them to the fascinating area of voice research and recording and analyzing and isolating questions that are possible to answer. Working with young people is wonderful, and many of them ask for a position as a doctoral student. So, that would be nice if I had a big grant.

A burning question is if, and under what conditions, the vocal tract sound is attacking the glottal airflow? It seems that singers have found a way to circumvent this danger. It is likely that some combinations of formant frequency and fundamental frequency ruin the control of the voice, and that of course is not acceptable in singing. You must be the master of the voice if you want to sing, so good singers must have found a way around this danger and what the trick is will be a nice to find out. And I think that may come in the future.

And then models of the vocal tract and the glottal voice source. That should be an important contribution but that may be taking some time.

More information about the voice source and how it varies, and what parameters of the voice source are reliably reflecting glottal adduction. I think glottal adduction is a key concept, because if you exaggerate it, you run into hyperfunctionality and then you are very likely to damage your voice. But we are not there yet. It is not possible to see in an unequivocal way from the flow glottogram what adduction is. With the enormous amounts of information we have about the voice source today it should be available in the near future.

18

Outside the Box

To start exploring the next best questions for a particular population.

C. Sapienza, PhD

C Sapienza, PhD: I just think that we need to continue to ask new questions. I would like to see the newer generation continue to ask hard experimental questions. I would like to challenge them to maintain tight experimental design, to encourage our group of researchers to be statistically mindful of the questions that they are asking.

Sometimes, I see reinvention of questions that have been answered twenty years ago. I would just like us to start exploring the next best questions for a particular population.

I. Titze, PhD: I am now convinced that good voice use is not only important for effective speech communication, but also for general health. If we were to use our larynx for more non-speech vocalization, such as singing, wailing, and calling, we would likely be healthier. Certain hormone productions are enhanced by vibrational stimuli. Loud sneezing, coughing, even occasional shouting, are probably a good thing.

So much emphasis in human communication has been on conversational-level speech. I believe that if speaking is all one does with the larynx, it may lose much of its capability. I have studied the larynxes of other mammals. They use a much wider range of pitch, loudness, and voice quality in their vocalizations. I think we are taking an evolutionarily step backwards by just speaking at conversational level.

There is an historical tradition of chanting: Sanskrit, Mongolian, Tuvan, Gregorian, to name a few. They all have a purpose beyond verbal communication. One of my PhD students is doing very early studies on the production of hormones by cells under tissue vibration that mimics vocalization.

R.J. Baken, PhD: The last several years have been pretty much devoted to pondering the ultimate utility of the theory of non-linear dynamics, a relatively new branch of mathematics. I've been incredibly frustrated. I've written and lectured a lot about it, some of my efforts technical and some hortatory. It is popularly known as the chaos theory, which is a bad name. Its popularity in the general public was spread by Gleick's book, but I got hooked into it when I read that its mathematical basis is mixed up with fractal geometry, invented by a guy named Benoit Mandelbrot, a pure mathematician (IBM researcher). He wrote a very important and very short paper that appeared in the journal *Science* titled 'How Long Is The Coast Of Britain?' which is probably one of the most famous mathematics paper of the 20th century, and it just stunned me with the conviction that it offered a way not only to quantify vocal irregularity but to reveal deeper aspects of its origins. In any case, chaos theory became chic, so there are a lot of people now tinkering with it, including many who haven't come to grips with its basic principles and – even more – with its basic mathematics. I've been unbelievably frustrated by my inability to convey the essential elements of chaos theory (in the context of vocal function) to many of my colleagues, or to convince them of its enormous explanatory (and ultimately clinical) potential. When I can, however, I soldier on.

How does this relate to jitter and shimmer? Jitter and shimmer purport to measure irregularity, but it's easy to show that they really don't. Chaos theory and fractal geometry, on the other hand, provide a means of quantifying unpredictability (unpredictability is irregularity) and of demonstrating inherent properties of an irregular signal that escape other approaches. Philip Lieberman (and Clarence Simon before him) had a potentially good idea, but I don't believe it's panned out for voice specialists. It's time to move on.

———

R. C. Scherer, PhD: What would you do with an open-ended, perfect grant?

It's in the line of what Jim Gould was about and The Voice Foundation is still all about. I would like to a see a multidisciplinary project going on that would combine basic science through performance science.

It would be a huge project that dealt with advancing the knowledge of voice production across disciplines, research on all aspects of voice, tissues to modeling, bench studies to self-expression, mechanics to psychology, surgery to the stage, and be involved after that with the dissemination of new knowledge, new techniques, new theories, and new and effective approaches to changing the voice in therapy and the studio, etc. There are just a thousand things to do, and the best way to deal with that is to get a hundred people together who are the best in the field, and create a synergistic project area.

There have been larger funded, multi-institutional grants through NIH over the years. Our P60 grant, with Ingo in the lead, dealt with multiple projects, training, and dissemination. With enough funding (a great deal of funding), it would be possible to form a global consortium of the best minds and labs, to strengthen those labs, improve research education, and collectively tackle well-defined questions to solve immediate and future needs in voice across all voice professions.

———

J. Rubin, MD: I think The Voice Foundation should continue to reach out to scientists, and I think it should perhaps be looking at working with associated disciplines, because as we try to recreate a larynx, or restore vocal function, we need to work with teams who are doing similar work in such disparate areas as say cardiac arrhythmia or ligamentous injury of the knee. The orthopedic surgeons, in particular, are far ahead of us in reconstruction of joints and ligaments and we need to work with them. The larynx is a biomechanical structure with complex neural and hormonal underpinnings. We need to share our knowledge with these other groups so we can all work together. This is something that Jim Gould recognized all those years ago, and is as germane today as it was forty-plus years ago when The Voice Foundation was new.

———

C. Sapienza, PhD: What's going on right now that I think is really exciting, is this whole area of simulation training. We haven't done that much of it in speech pathology, we're starting to dabble in it.

It's been going on in the nursing field for a little while, using mannequin-based simulation virtual patient portfolios that you can create and manipulate and students can learn from. You can train a student in patient care, intubation, feeding and swallowing, and really look at the physiologic response of the body through simulation now.

You can show students three-dimensional anatomy that has been recreated from cadaver specimen. You could never do that. You could only teach them in a two-dimensional way. Teaching in a three-dimensional way is huge.

To think the high-speed stroboscopy has taught us so much about things that we thought were going on, with regard to vibratory mechanics with particular disorders. You're able to develop new theories of vibratory pattern and with the model in different conditions, because with the model you can be very specific about the biomechanics of vibration, and high-speed film has brought us that. I think those are some of the major things that I've seen go on in the last five or six years.

New Ways to Hear

R. H. Colton, PhD: I've always been interested in the disconnect between what you see acoustically – the signal – and what people hear. We, the scientific community, have done a lot of work over the years trying to look at that, and still have not quite answered the basic questions. But we are making progress. What the relationship is between the perceptual world, what you hear in the clinic, on the stage, or in the opera house, and what we see in the physical world when people are producing that. In some cases, I think we don't have the techniques to do that yet. Over the years I've been doing this, it has happened a lot. We don't have the techniques to do something, then a few years later, bongo!, something has come out.

I think it is a question of working at it, finding the techniques that will help us to draw a better relationship between what's coming out of a person's mouth in the physical world, and what the listener hears. That involves the ear, so we really have to take a careful look at what our friends in hearing science are doing, which we do. But perhaps not well enough yet. Or perhaps they may not be interested in what we are doing. So we need to get a collaborative arrangement with them.

That's always been my interest over the years, of how we can relate the two. Sometimes we find these differences and it doesn't make any difference to the patient who is producing it. It is a big area.

R. T. Sataloff, MD, DMA: When I first got involved in laryngology in the late 1970s to very early 1980s, there were three voice labs in the United States. Now there are several hundred voice labs pretty much everywhere where there is serious laryngology. Their level of sophistication varies, but many people are trying to do something to document and quantify voice signals. That's happened over the last thirty years. However, I think that everything that we have is intrinsically deficient and obsolete, and that our whole paradigm and instrumentation needs to change. So, I think that everything we're doing is better than nothing, but not nearly as good as it should be. We need a whole new paradigm.

I think we need to get a group together that involves people with expertise in aerospace signal detection technology and self-educating computers to develop a whole new approach that merges technological measurements with the human ability to hear, so that we can train instruments to be as sensitive as our ears. At the moment, they are not.

We need signal detection technology that's much more sophisticated than a microphone and a mechanical piece of equipment that analyzes components of an acoustic signal, like the kind of signal detection technology that aerospace experts use to look for meaningful signals coming from other planets in the midst of space noise. Then, we need to run the signals through very complex computers and teach them what they're hearing, just as we teach ourselves through perceptual training, in order to get computers that are at least as acoustically and analytically sensitive as the human ear. But that's my opinion.

The technology is there. It's a matter of finding and getting the people who have the right skills and the right interests together in the right place with the right funding.

19

Broadening the Circle

> Everything starts at a higher knowledge level at each meeting.
>
> R.T. Sataloff, MD, DMA

R.T. Sataloff, MD, DMA: The Symposia have changed through a natural and predictable evolution. The science of voice – clinical and research – has developed dramatically greater knowledge, hence the people who attended the Symposia, and the people who present at the Symposia know more as a basic knowledge base than the most sophisticated and informed of us had any clue about, even with all of us combined, during the early Symposia. Therefore, everything starts at a higher knowledge level at each meeting than it did even a year or two before, and unrecognizably so compared with a decade or two before.

Our ability to define questions of scientific interest and clinical relevance has gotten much better. The specificity of those questions has gotten more incisive. And we are coming to the point at which we are ready for new inspiration by bringing in research experts in other disciplines who have never been involved with the Symposia or with voice research before, and getting them involved to identify and clarify the issues that we haven't recognized in an articulate fashion so far. For example, world-class aerodynamicists, potentially more sophisticated experts in nonlinear dynamics, and people in other disciplines. As that happens, the Symposia will continue to remain vital and cutting edge.

I am committed to broadening the circle, and that's what we have done since the beginning. It's time to step back, take a fresh and unbiased look, and widen it again.

Appendices

The Voice Foundation 2015 Board of Directors

Robert Thayer Sataloff	Chairman
Stuart Orsher	President
Michael S. Benninger	Vice-President
Mary Hawkshaw	Secretary
Brian P. Flaherty	General Counsel
Michael M. Johns, III	Chairman, Advisory Board

Martina Arroyo
Harolyn Blackwell
Claudia Catania
Jennifer Creed
Gwen Korovin
Renata Scotto
Justice Sandra Schultz Newman
Michael Sheehan
George Shirley
Caren J. Sokolow
Diana Soviero

www.voicefoundation,org

2015 Advisory Board

Michael M. Johns, III, MD, Chairman
Mona Abaza, MD
Jean Abitbol, MD
R.J. Baken, PhD
Mara Behlau, PhD
Diane M. Bless, PhD
Daniel R. Boone, PhD
William S. Brown, PhD
Thomas Carroll, MD
Raymond H. Colton, PhD
Kathleen T. Cox, PhD
Pamela Davis, PhD
Molly Erickson, MM, PhD
Charles N. Ford, MD, FACS
Adrian Fourcin, PhD
Glendon M. Gardner, MD
Abdul-Latif Hamdan, MD, FACS
Mary Hawkshaw, RN, BSN, CORLN
Christian Herbst, PhD
Shigeru Hirano, MD, PhD
Hajime Hirose, MD
Norman D. Hogikyan, MD
Harry Hollien, PhD
David Howard, PhD, BS
Jack J. Jiang, MD, PhD
Joel Kahane, PhD
Michael Kalisman, MD
Gwen S. Korovin, MD
Denis C. Lafreniere, MD, FACS

Charles R. Larson, PhD
Jeannette L. LoVetri
Christy L. Ludlow, PhD
Nicolas E. Maragos, MD
Albert Merati, MD
David Meyer, DM
John Michel, PhD
Claudio F. Milstein, PhD
Thomas Murry, PhD
Robert H. Ossoff, DMD, MD
Michael Pitman, MD
Paulo Pontes, MD
Lisa S. Popeil, MFA
Adam Rubin, MD
Wallace Rubin, MD
Lucille S. Rubin, PhD
John S. Rubin, MD, FACS, FRCS
Ronald C. Scherer, PhD
Rahul Shrivastav, PhD
Donna Snow, MFA
Nancy Pearl Solomon, PhD
Johan Sundberg, PhD
Jan Švec, PhD
Sten Ternström, PhD
Harvey M. Tucker, MD, FACS
Peter J. Watson, PhD
Peak Woo, MD
Gayle Woodson, MD
Edwin Yiu, PhD

Voice Education Research Awareness (Vera) Award Recipients

Geraldine Dietz Fox 1990
Enrico Manca 1991
Anthony Quinn 1993
Dan Rather 1993
Anna Moffo Sarnoff 1993
Adele Warden Paxson 1993
John R. Stafford 1994
Alan King 1994
Phyllis Curtin 1994
Rotan E. Lee 1994
David W. Brewer, MD 1995
Malcolm Poindexter 1995
Brian McDonough, MD 1996
Licia Albanese 1997
Berle Schiller 1997
Leon Fassler 1998
Sherrill Milnes 1998
Grace Bumbry 1999
Matina Horner 1999
George Shirley 1999
Richard Leech 2000
David Bradley 2000
Jack Klugman 2001
Dame Julie Andrews 2002
Samuel Katz 2002
Renata Scotto 2003
Constantine Papadakis, PhD 2003
Robert Driver 2004
Aprile Millo 2004
Teddy Pendergrass 2004
James Gerlach 2005
Giorgio Tozzi 2005

Shirley Verrett 2005
Martina Arroyo 2006
Richard Miller, PhD 2006
Ben Vereen 2006
David Bradley 2000
Jack Klugman 2001
Dame Julie Andrews 2002
Harolyn Blackwell 2007
Robert Goulet 2007
Marni Nixon 2007
Justice Sandra Schultz Newman 2007
Claudia Catania 2008
Lisa Thomas-Laury 2008
Manuel N. Stamatakis 2008
Glen Campbell 2009
Charles Dutoit 2009
Ruth Ann Swenson 2009
Richard Homan 2010
Peter Nero 2010
Paul Plishka 2010
Barry Bittman 2011
Diane Rehm 2011
Diana Soviero 2011
Terry Stewart 2011
Frederica von Stade 2012
Byron Janis 2012
Vy Higginsen 2013
Susanne Mentzer 2013
Roberta Flack 2014
Denise Graves 2014
Dolora Zajick 2015
Stacy Keach 2015

Raymond and Beverly Sackler Award Recipients

Helen Hayes 1988
Walter Cronkite 1989
James Earl Jones 1990
Jessica Tandy 1991
C. Everett Koop 1992
Jack Klugman 1995
Nancy Snyderman, MD 1999
Celeste Holm 2000
Terry Gross 2002

Tony Randall 2003
Justice Sandra Schultz Newman 2007
Bobby Rydell 2011
Danny Aiello 2012
Michael Sheehan 2012
Anthony Lacuria 2013
Dr John 2013
Bootsy Collins 2014
Joel Grey 2015

Wilbur James Gould Award

Anna Moffo Sarnoff 1996
Sadanand Singh, PhD 2001

Robert T. Sataloff 2007

Tony Randall Award

Eli Wallach 2008

Hamdan International Presentation Award

Laura Enflo 2012
Christian Herbst 2013

Edwin Yiu 2014

Honored Symposium Master Class Teachers

Renata Scotto 1984
John Moriarty 1985
John Wustman 1986
Anna Moffo 1987
Phyllis Curtin 1988
Max Rudolf 1989
Frank Guerarra 1990
Craig Ruttenberg 1991
Barbara Silverstein 1992
Harold Evans 1993
Phyllis Curtin 1994
George Shirley 1995
Ruth Falcon 1996
Cynthia Hoffmann 1997
Sherrill Milnes 1998
Leslie Guinn 1999

Claudia Catania 2000
Tito Capobianco 2001
Susan Ashbaker 2002
Sharon Sweet 2003
Christofer Macatsoris 2004
Shirley Verrett 2005
Martina Arroyo 2006
Susan Ashbaker 2007
Katherine Ciesinski 2008
John Burrows 2009
Harolyn Blackwell 2010
Diana Soviero 2011
Frederica von Stade 2012
Susanne Mentzer 2013
Denyce Graves 2014
Dolora Zajick 2015

G. Paul Moore Lecturers

G. Paul Moore 1981
Hans von Leden 1982
Friedrich Brodnitz 1983
Harry Hollien 1984
John A. Kirchner 1985
Henry J. Rubin 1986
Minoru Hirano 1987
David W. Brewer 1988
Johan Sundberg 1989
Oskar Kleinsasser 1990
Wilbur J. Gould 1991
Ingo R. Titze 1992
Harvey M. Tucker 1993
Robert T. Sataloff 1994
Richard Miller 1995
Nobuhiko Isshiki 1996
Aatto Sonninen 1997
Steven Gray 1998

Joel Kahane 1999
Jean Westerman Gregg 2000
Daniel R. Boone 2001
Ronald C. Scherer 2002
Charles Ford 2003
R.J. Baken 2004
Janina Casper 2005
Christy Ludlow 2006
Jean Abitbol 2007
Diane Bless 2008
Michael S. Benninger 2009
Bonnie Raphael 2010
Katherin Verdolini Abbott 2011
Peak Woo 2012
Thomas Murry 2013
Gayle Woodson 2014
Brenda Smith 2015

Quintana Voice Research Award Recipients

Kenzo Ishizaka 1989
Gunnar Fant 1990
Ingo R. Titze 1991
Kenneth Stevens 1992
Martin Rothenberg 1993
Jan Gauffin 1995
Aatto Sonninen 1997
Donald Childers 2000

Adrian Fourcin 2004
Masayuki Sawashima 2006
Johan Sundberg 2008
Harm Schutte 2010
Kiyoshi Honda 2012
Fariborz Alipour 2014
Ulrich Eysholdt 2015

Sataloff Young Investigators Award Recipients

Heather Shaw Bonilha 2009
Rosiane Yamasaki 2010
Satoshi Ohno 2011

Matthew Hoffman 2012
Aaron Johnson 2013
Jessica Sofranco Kisenwether 2014

Van L. Lawrence Fellowship Recipients

Lois Yadeau 1991
Raquel Cortina 1992
Karen Peeler 1993
Lynelle F. Wiens 1993
Kenneth Bozeman 1994
Janette Ogg 1994
Thomas Houser 1995
Sue W. Snyder 1995
Ruth Golden 1996
Freda Herseth 1997
 Marvin Keenze 1998
Kathleen Wilson 1998
Jeannette Lovetri 1999
Steven Austin 1999
Brenda Smith 2000
Meribeth Bunch 2001
Jan Prokop 2002
Katherine Eberle 2003
Norman Spivey 2003
Lynn Helding 2005
 John Nix 2006
Kathryn Barnes-Burroughs 2007
Margaret Baroody 2008
Donald Bell 2009
David Meyer 2010
Brian Gill 2011
Kari Ragan 2012
Bonnie Draina 2013
Katherine Osborne, 2014
Filipa Martins Baptista Lã, 2015

About the Author

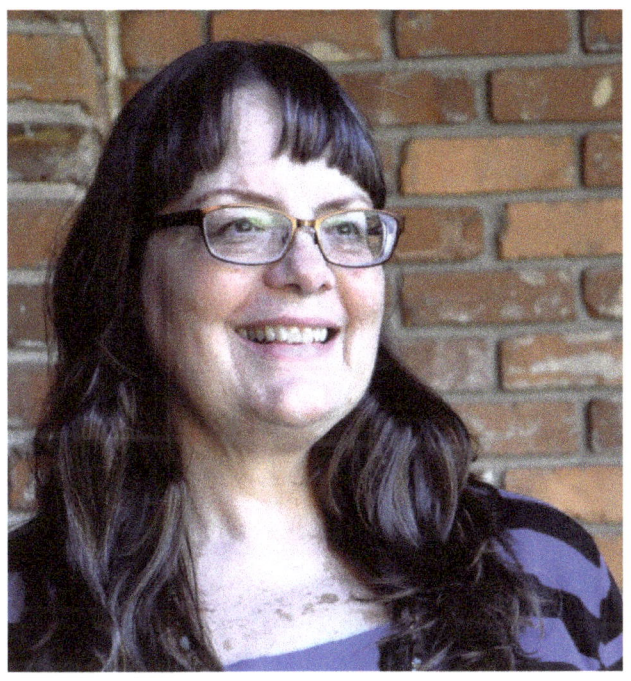

Picture: Dana Statton

After an extensive performance path beginning with folk and church music, passing through the baroque, concert work and over fifty recitals, landing squarely in Wagner, Strauss and 20th – 21st century opera, with over a hundred roles on major stages, Martha Howe began teaching Voice, Acting While Singing, and Breathing in a Musicals school in Vienna, before returning to the US in 2007. Her stylistically wide-ranging studio includes Skype students in Europe and the US, and she is coaching business people on their presentation skills.

Attending her first Symposium in 2011 was a revelatory experience. She found it fascinating to discover the science behind the vocal traditions. Vocally and technically, things were coming full circle.

In 1907, Maude Douglas Tweedy stopped her concert career and began to work with Dr Frank E. Miller, the leading laryngologist in New York City. By 1912, she had her regular studio of professional singers and was also what would be known today as Dr Miller's Singing Health Specialist, working with his patients to clear vocal injuries and retraining them to prevent future injuries. Mme Tweedy died in 1985, at the age of 98, after 70 years of teaching.

Martha was one of Tweedy's last students. She then worked with master teacher Jane Randolph (presently at the San Francisco Conservatory) who inherited and refined Mme Tweedy's technique. So it is not surprising that the science has only supported and clarified, never contradicted, this technique.

Martha has been writing for publication since 1998, and received a Master of Arts in Literature through the British Open University in 2008.

You are invited to visit her website: marthahowe.com and her blog: groundedvocalfreedom.wordpress.com.

www.ingramcontent.com/pod-product-compliance
Lightning Source LLC
Chambersburg PA
CBHW061140230426
43663CB00027B/2987